AF879402

The Vegan Voyage

Pasquel Jordan-McLeod

Published by JourNique Publishing Group
United States

ISBN: 978-0-9795586-2-7

Contents

Setting Sail on The Vegan Voyage

Welcome aboard *The Vegan Voyage*, a journey that explores the profound connection between what we eat and how we live. This book is more than just a collection of recipes; it's a compass guiding us back to the roots of true nourishment. In a world where our dietary choices have drifted far from what was once intended to sustain and heal us, *The Vegan Voyage* invites you to embark on a path of rediscovery.

As we navigate through the pages, we'll explore how modern eating habits, filled with processed and toxin-laden foods, have led to a rise in health issues that affect us earlier in life than ever before. But this voyage is not just about what we leave behind—it's about embracing a new way of living, one that celebrates the vibrant, life-giving foods that nature intended for us.

On this journey, you'll discover that plant-based eating isn't about restriction or sacrifice; it's about abundance, creativity, and the joy of nurturing your body with foods that are as delicious as they are nourishing. Each recipe is a stop on our voyage, offering a taste of the diverse and flavorful world of vegan cuisine.

So, whether you're a seasoned vegan or just beginning to explore this lifestyle, *The Vegan Voyage* is your guide to a healthier, more compassionate way of eating. Together, we'll chart a course toward vibrant health, environmental sustainability, and a deep connection with the food that fuels us.

Let's set sail on this adventure and discover the rich, satisfying world of vegan living—one meal at a time.

Reclaiming Health: The Path to Vibrant Living

Whenever I tell a friend or family member that I have converted to a plant-based diet, their first response is often, "How do you get your protein?" The Western misconception that only meat contains the protein necessary for a healthy diet couldn't be farther from the truth. In reality, there is an abundance of plant-based foods that are rich in protein.

For instance, legumes such as lentils, chickpeas, and black beans are excellent sources of protein. Nuts and seeds, including almonds, chia seeds, and hemp seeds, are not only protein-packed but also provide healthy fats and essential nutrients. Whole grains like quinoa, farro, and bulgur offer substantial protein content along with fiber and minerals. Even vegetables such as spinach, broccoli, and Brussels sprouts contribute to daily protein intake.

Fruits like guava and apricots, while not as protein-dense as legumes or grains, still contain a noteworthy amount. By diversifying your diet with these plant-based proteins, you can easily meet your nutritional needs while enjoying a variety of delicious, wholesome foods. It's important to note that a plant-based diet can be healthy when well-balanced, providing all essential nutrients. However, individuals need to pay attention to getting a variety of plant-based foods to ensure they meet their nutritional needs, especially for nutrients like vitamin B12, iron, calcium, and omega-3 fatty acids, which are less abundant in plant foods.

As with any diet, the key to optimal health is making thoughtful and informed choices, considering individual health goals, nutritional needs, and preferences. Consulting with a healthcare professional or registered dietitian can provide personalized guidance for adopting a plant-based diet that meets one's specific health requirements.

Far too often, there's a prevailing misconception that a plant-based diet equates to dull and uninspiring meals. This couldn't be farther from reality. The fascinating world of plant-based cuisine is an artistic canvas waiting to be explored. It's a realm where you can fuse a diverse array of ingredients and culinary techniques to create not just nourishing but also incredibly delicious dishes.

In this realm, you'll discover a vast spectrum of fruits, vegetables, legumes, grains, nuts, and seeds, each offering its unique flavors and textures. You can delve into the rich tapestry of global cuisines, uncovering exotic tastes and culinary traditions from different corners of the world.

Don't underestimate the power of herbs and spices, either. They are the unsung heroes of plant-based cooking, capable of transforming ordinary ingredients into extraordinary feasts for the senses. With the right seasoning, you can craft dishes that burst with complex and harmonious flavors.

Plant-based proteins, such as tofu, tempeh, and legumes, are versatile ingredients that can mimic the textures and tastes of animal-based proteins. They allow you to recreate your favorite dishes without compromising on flavor or nutrition.

The creative possibilities are boundless! You can roast, grill, sauté, stir-fry, or bake your way to culinary excellence, each technique imparting a unique character to your dishes.

For those who crave the comfort of dairy, there's a burgeoning selection of plant-based alternatives to explore, from almond milk to cashew cheese, offering creamy textures and delightful tastes.

And when that occasional craving for indulgence strikes, you can find plant-based alternatives to favorite junk foods like burgers, pizzas, and ice cream that deliver all the satisfaction without the guilt.

The vibrant and nutrient-rich nature of plant-based ingredients make your meals not only delicious but also visually appealing and nourishing. Beyond the culinary pleasures, a plant-based diet carries significant health and environmental benefits, serving as a rewarding choice for your well-being and the planet.

In essence, the world of plant-based cuisine is a treasure trove of flavors, textures, and culinary adventures waiting for you to explore. It's a journey that promises not just delicious meals but also a healthier, more sustainable way of eating.

I made the decision to write this book with the primary aim of sharing a collection of healthy and delectable recipes that have been tried and tested by my own family. Throughout these pages, I hope to offer you a glimpse into the wonderful world of flavorful, nutritious cooking that has brought joy to my household. Each recipe included has been carefully crafted to not only tantalize your taste buds but also provide nourishment and well-being. I look forward to taking you on this culinary journey, where you can discover the same satisfaction and delight that my loved ones have experienced through these dishes.

Break of Day: Nourishing Vegan Breakfasts

The idea that "breakfast is the most important meal of the day" has been a common belief for a long time. It suggests that having a morning meal carries significant benefits. It marks the end of the overnight fast, providing your body with the energy it needs after a period without food. Breakfast can also enhance your alertness, concentration, and cognitive functions, which is especially valuable for students and people with demanding daily schedules.

Breakfast offers an opportunity to intake essential nutrients like vitamins, minerals, and fiber, which might be lacking if you skip it. Some research even suggests that a nutritious breakfast can help with weight management by reducing overall calorie consumption during the day. Additionally, breakfast can play a role in stabilizing blood sugar levels, preventing energy fluctuations.

Establishing a regular eating routine, which includes breakfast, can also promote healthier eating habits. It is crucial to acknowledge that everyone's body functions differently. Some individuals may not feel hungry in the morning and may prefer to eat later in the day. Ultimately, what matters most is maintaining a balanced and nutritious diet that suits your unique needs and preferences, regardless of when you choose to have your meals.

Switching to a vegan or plant-based diet means saying goodbye to eggs and other animal-based products. Our culture has grown so accustomed to classics like eggs and bacon for breakfast that it can be quite a challenge to reimagine our morning meals. When my family first embarked on our vegan journey, we faced this very hurdle. However, with some experimentation and culinary exploration, we've not only overcome it but also discovered a range of delightful breakfast options that we absolutely love.

Oat-Standing Beginnings: Perfecting Baked Oatmeal

The first breakfast recipe I'm going to share is baked oatmeal. I chose this as the opening recipe because it was the very first dish I made when I began my vegan journey. This warm, comforting dish quickly became a staple in my kitchen, offering a delicious and nutritious way to start the day.

Over the years, I've experimented with various ingredients and techniques, perfecting it to suit my tastes and preferences. Now, it's a versatile recipe that can be customized with your favorite fruits, nuts, and spices, making it a beloved breakfast option for any season.

Baked oatmeal is one of my family's beloved go-to breakfasts. It's not only delicious but also quick and simple to prepare. What I love most about it is its versatility – there are numerous variations to explore. Plus, if you have a hectic schedule, you can make a batch of baked oatmeal in advance and keep it in the refrigerator for a few days, making mornings much more manageable.

Baked oatmeal is just the tip of the iceberg when it comes to delicious vegan breakfast options. There's a vast world of morning meals waiting to be explored. Since seven is often considered a number of completion, here are seven mouthwatering breakfast ideas to tantalize your taste buds. I'm excited to share my perfected version with you, hoping it becomes a favorite in your home as well.

Baked Oatmeal

Ingredients

- 2 cups 100% Whole grain Organic rolled oats
- 1/2 cup chopped nuts (e.g., almonds, walnuts, or pecans)
- 1/2 cup dried fruit (e.g., raisins, cranberries, or chopped dates)
- 1 teaspoon aluminum free baking powder
- 1/2 teaspoon cinnamon
- 1/4 teaspoon salt
- 2 cups organic plant-based milk (e.g., almond milk, or oat milk)
- 1/4 cup organic maple syrup or monk fruit sweetener
- 1 teaspoon vanilla extract
- 1 ripe banana, mashed
- 1/2 cup applesauce or mashed apples

Optional toppings: sliced bananas, berries, or additional nuts and seeds

Instructions

1. Preheat your oven to 350°F (175°C). Grease a baking dish (approximately 8x8 inches) or line it with parchment paper for easy cleanup.
2. In a mixing bowl, combine the rolled oats, chopped nuts, dried fruit, baking powder, cinnamon, and salt. Mix well to evenly distribute the ingredients.
3. In another bowl, whisk together the plant-based milk, maple syrup, vanilla extract, mashed banana, and applesauce.
4. Pour the wet mixture into the dry mixture and stir until everything is well combined.
5. Pour the oatmeal mixture into the prepared baking dish, spreading it out evenly.
6. If desired, add optional toppings such as sliced bananas, berries, or additional nuts and seeds.
7. Bake in the preheated oven for 30-35 minutes or until the top is golden brown, and the oatmeal is set. The baking time may vary slightly depending on your oven, so keep an eye on it.
8. Remove the baked oatmeal from the oven and let it cool for a few minutes before serving.

9. Serve warm slices of vegan baked oatmeal with your favorite plant-based yogurt, extra fruit, or a drizzle of organic maple syrup, if desired.

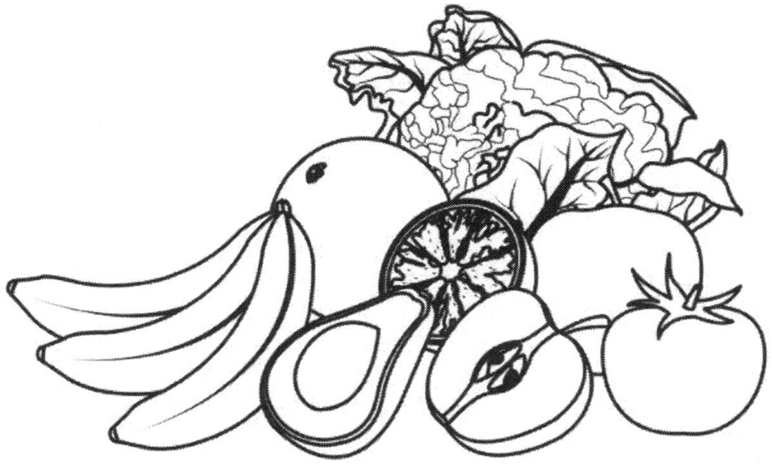

Gluten-Free Goodness: Hearty Breakfast Burritos to Start Your Day

This next recipe I'm excited to share is a hearty breakfast burrito. This filling and nutritious meal is perfect for starting your day with a burst of energy. Packed with wholesome ingredients, it's a delicious way to fuel your morning while sticking to a plant-based diet.

In addition to avoiding meat, I also steer clear of foods that aren't clean. My rule of thumb is simple: if you can't pronounce an ingredient, chances are it shouldn't be consumed, especially not frequently. Opting for clean, whole foods ensures that you're nourishing your body with the best nature has to offer.

When possible, always choose the organic option. Organic foods are grown without synthetic pesticides and fertilizers, which means they're better for your health and the environment. Be sure to use organic fresh vegetables and organic whole grains whenever possible. Reading food labels is crucial to understanding what you're putting into your body. Avoid foods with added sugars, unhealthy fats, preservatives, and artificial additives. Look for foods with short ingredient lists that feature recognizable, whole-food components.

This breakfast burrito embodies these principles, combining fresh organic vegetables, organic whole grains, and organic protein-rich beans. It's not only a tasty and satisfying meal but also a clean and wholesome choice you can feel good about. Enjoy this burrito as a nutritious start to your day, knowing you're making choices that support your health and well-being.

Breakfast Burrito

Ingredients

- 1 cup cooked and mashed organic sweet potatoes
- 1 tablespoon olive oil
- 1/2 cup diced organic bell peppers (any color)
- 1/2 cup diced organic onions
- 1/2 cup organic black beans, drained and rinsed
- 1/2 teaspoon organic ground cumin
- 1/2 teaspoon organic chili powder
- Pink himalayan salt and pepper to taste
- 4 large almond flour tortillas
- 1 cup organic spinach or kale leaves, washed and chopped
- 1 organic avocado, sliced
- 1/4 cup organic salsa (optional)
- Hot sauce (optional)

Instructions

Step 1: Mash Sweet Potatoes

Ingredients:

- 2 large sweet potatoes
- 2 tablespoons olive oil
- Salt to taste
- Pepper to taste
- 1/2 teaspoon ground cumin (optional)
- 1/2 teaspoon smoked paprika (optional)

Instructions:

1. Preheat Oven:
    - Preheat your oven to 400°F (200°C).

2. Prepare Sweet Potatoes:
    - Wash and peel the sweet potatoes.
    - Cut them into evenly sized cubes, about 1-inch pieces.
3. Roast Sweet Potatoes:
    - Place the sweet potato cubes on a baking sheet lined with parchment paper.
    - Drizzle with olive oil and sprinkle with salt, pepper, ground cumin, and smoked paprika (if using).
    - Toss to coat the sweet potatoes evenly.
    - Spread them out in a single layer on the baking sheet.
4. Bake:
    - Bake in the preheated oven for 25-30 minutes, or until the sweet potatoes are tender and easily pierced with a fork.
    - Stir halfway through the cooking time to ensure even roasting.
5. Mash:

Once the sweet potatoes are done, transfer them to a large mixing bowl.

Use a potato masher or fork to mash the sweet potatoes until smooth and creamy.

Taste and adjust seasoning with more salt and pepper if needed.

6. Set Aside:

Set the mashed sweet potatoes aside while you prepare the other components of the breakfast burrito.

Your mashed sweet potatoes are now ready to be added to your delicious Organic Gluten-Free Vegan Breakfast Burritos!

1. Heat the olive oil in a large skillet over medium heat.

2. Add the diced bell peppers and onions to the skillet. Sauté for 3-4 minutes or until they start to soften.

3. Stir in the mashed sweet potatoes, ground cumin, chili powder, salt, and pepper. Cook for an additional 5-7 minutes, or until everything is heated through and well combined.

4. Add the black beans to the sweet potato mixture and cook for an additional 2 minutes to warm them.

5. Warm the whole-grain tortillas in a dry skillet or microwave for about 15 seconds to make them pliable.

6. Lay out each tortilla on a clean surface.

7. Place a generous scoop of the sweet potato and black bean mixture onto each tortilla, spreading it out evenly down the center.

8. Add a handful of chopped spinach or kale leaves on top of the filling.

9. Add a few slices of avocado to each burrito.

10. If desired, spoon salsa and hot sauce over the fillings for extra flavor.

11. To fold the burritos, first fold in the sides of the tortilla, then roll up from the bottom to create a secure wrap.

12. Place each finished burrito seam-side down on a plate.

13. Your Vegan Breakfast Burritos are ready to enjoy! Serve them immediately, or wrap them in foil for a portable breakfast on the go.

Savor the deliciousness of these Organic Gluten-Free Vegan Breakfast Burritos, featuring a flavorful sweet potato and black bean filling, fresh veggies, and creamy avocado. They're a nutritious and satisfying way to start your day, whether you're at home or on the move.

Choosing gluten-free options is not only beneficial for those with celiac disease or gluten intolerance but also for minimizing gluten-related ailments. Many conditions, such as irritable bowel syndrome (IBS), chronic fatigue, and certain autoimmune diseases, are associated with gluten. In my own experience, removing gluten from my son's diet significantly reduced the symptoms associated with his autism, leading to notable improvements in his overall well-being.

These burritos are versatile and customizable. Add your favorite toppings like diced tomatoes, vegan cheese, or plant-based sour cream to suit your taste preferences. Enjoy a delicious, nutritious breakfast that supports a healthy lifestyle and caters to specific dietary needs.

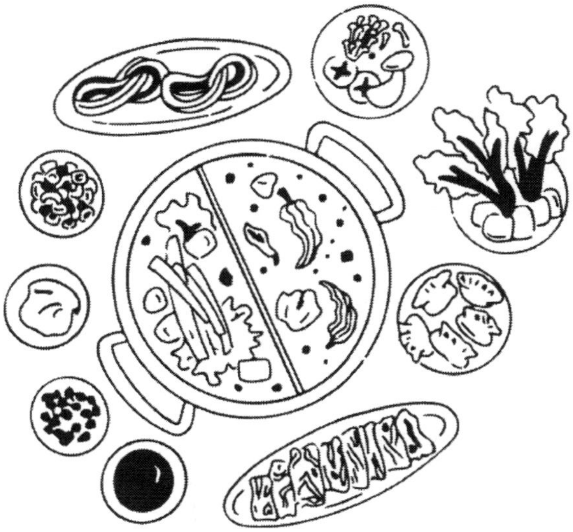

Morning Bliss: Deliciously Nutty Fruit Smoothie Bowl

When making smoothies, achieving a perfectly smooth and creamy texture is crucial. This means investing in a high-quality blender that can handle the task efficiently. A good blender ensures that your fruits and other ingredients are thoroughly blended, providing the ideal consistency for your smoothie bowl.

I learned this lesson from personal experience. Initially, I opted for cheaper, lower-quality blenders, which often struggled to blend ingredients properly. Due to daily use, these blenders broke down quickly, forcing me to replace them every year. This cycle of repeat purchases was both frustrating and costly. It became clear that spending a bit more on a durable, high-performance blender was a wise investment in both my kitchen and my health.

Starting your day with a smoothie bowl packed with fresh fruits offers a range of health benefits. Fruits provide essential vitamins, minerals, and antioxidants that support overall well-being. Here are five fruits that you might include in your smoothie bowl and what they're known for:

- **Blueberries:** Blueberries are renowned for their high antioxidant content, particularly anthocyanins, which help combat oxidative stress and inflammation. This makes them beneficial for brain health, potentially improving memory and cognitive function while reducing the risk of chronic diseases like heart disease and cancer.

- **Strawberries:** Strawberries are rich in vitamin C, an essential nutrient that supports the immune system and promotes healthy skin. They also contain manganese, which aids in bone health and metabolism. The antioxidants in strawberries have anti-inflammatory properties that help reduce the risk of chronic illnesses.

- **Raspberries:** Raspberries are packed with dietary fiber, which aids in digestion and helps maintain healthy blood sugar levels. The high fiber content supports heart health by reducing cholesterol levels and improving overall cardiovascular function. They also offer a range of vitamins and antioxidants that contribute to overall health.

- **Bananas:** Bananas are a fantastic source of potassium, which is crucial for maintaining heart health, regulating blood pressure, and supporting proper muscle function. They also provide a quick source of natural energy, making them an excellent choice for a morning boost. Additionally, bananas contain vitamin B6, which supports brain health and helps regulate mood.
- **Kiwi:** Kiwi is loaded with vitamin C, which supports immune function, skin health, and overall vitality. It also contains dietary fiber that aids digestion and helps maintain a healthy gut. The antioxidants in kiwi, such as vitamin E and polyphenols, contribute to cellular health and help protect against chronic diseases.

This Fruit and Nut Smoothie Bowl combines these nutrient-dense fruits with the satisfying crunch of nuts, creating a delicious and wholesome breakfast. By investing in a quality blender and incorporating these fruits into your morning routine, you're not only enhancing the flavor of your smoothie bowl but also boosting your overall health and well-being.

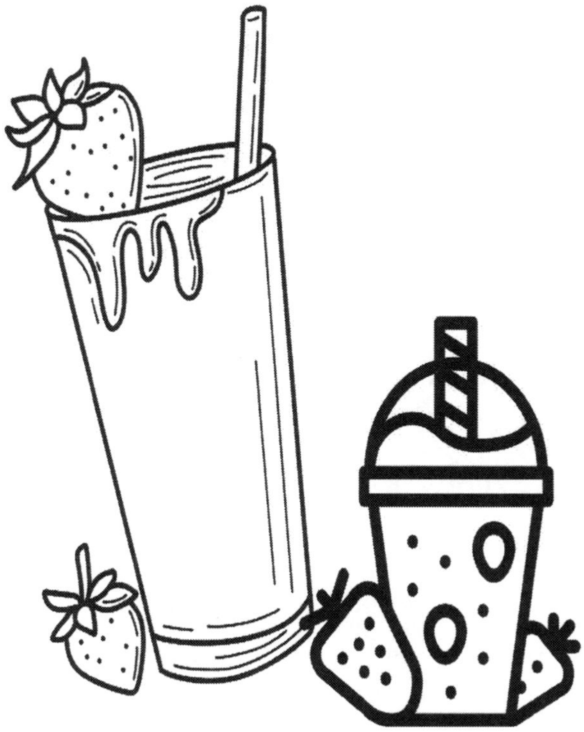

Fruit and Nut Smoothie Bowl

Ingredients

- 1 ripe banana, frozen
- 1 cup frozen mixed berries (strawberries, blueberries, raspberries)
- 1/2 cup plant-based yogurt (e.g., almond, coconut, or soy yogurt)
- 1/2 cup plant-based milk (e.g., almond, soy, or oat milk)
- 1 tablespoon maple syrup or another sweetener of your choice (optional)
- 1 teaspoon vanilla extract (optional)
- Sliced fresh fruits (e.g., kiwi, strawberries, and banana, for topping)
- Chopped nuts (e.g., almonds, walnuts, or pecans, for topping)
- Seeds (e.g., chia seeds, flax seeds, or pumpkin seeds, for topping)
- Granola (for topping)
- Coconut flakes (for topping)
- Fresh berries (for topping)
- Drizzle of honey or maple syrup (optional, for topping)

Instructions

1. In a blender, combine the frozen banana, frozen mixed berries, plant-based yogurt, plant-based milk, maple syrup (if using), and vanilla extract (if using).
2. Blend until smooth and creamy. You may need to pause and scrape down the sides of the blender to ensure everything is well combined.
3. Pour the smoothie mixture into a bowl.
4. Decorate your smoothie bowl with your favorite toppings. You can arrange sliced fresh fruits, nuts, seeds, granola, coconut flakes, fresh berries, or any other toppings you love.
5. If you prefer your smoothie bowl a bit sweeter, you can drizzle it with honey or maple syrup.
6. Grab a spoon and savor your colorful and nutritious smoothie bowl. Mix the toppings into the smoothie base as you enjoy each delicious bite.

Indulge in the delightful flavors and textures of this Fruit and Nut Smoothie Bowl. It's not just a feast for the eyes but also a wholesome way to fuel your day with essential nutrients and energy.

Customize it to your liking with your favorite fruits, nuts, and seeds for a breakfast that's both satisfying and refreshing.

This smoothie bowl recipe includes honey, a natural sweetener that adds a touch of richness. However, it's important to recognize that honey is not considered vegan. Honey is produced by bees, and the process of harvesting it can sometimes be detrimental to their well-being. The collection of honey often involves practices that may disturb or harm bee colonies, and for those committed to a vegan lifestyle, these practices are a significant concern. Additionally, the commercial honey industry can contribute to environmental issues related to large-scale bee farming.

For a vegan-friendly alternative, organic maple syrup is an excellent choice. Derived from the sap of sugar maple trees, organic maple syrup is not only vegan but also free from synthetic pesticides and fertilizers. Here's a closer look at the pros and cons of both sweeteners:

- Organic Maple Syrup:
    - **Pros:**
        - **Vegan-Friendly:** Maple syrup is a plant-based sweetener, making it suitable for those avoiding animal products.
        - **Natural and Clean:** Organic maple syrup is produced without synthetic chemicals, offering a cleaner option for those seeking natural ingredients.
        - **Nutritional Benefits:** It contains beneficial minerals such as manganese, zinc, and calcium, which support various bodily functions. It also has antioxidants that may help fight inflammation.
        - **Flavor Profile:** It has a rich, unique flavor that adds depth and complexity to recipes.
    - **Cons:**
        - **Cost:** Organic maple syrup is typically more expensive than conventional sweeteners.
        - **Flavor:** Its distinct taste may not be suitable for every recipe or personal preference.
- **Honey:**
    - **Pros:**
        - **Natural Sweetness:** Honey offers a pleasant, natural sweetness and has a variety of flavors depending on the floral source.
        - **Potential Health Benefits:** Honey contains antioxidants and has been traditionally used for its antimicrobial properties.
    - **Cons:**
        - **Not Vegan:** The use of honey is incompatible with vegan diets due to concerns

about animal welfare and the environmental impact of commercial beekeeping.

- **Ethical and Environmental Issues:** Honey production can sometimes involve practices that negatively impact bee health and biodiversity. The commercial honey industry also contributes to issues like habitat loss and monoculture farming.

By opting for organic maple syrup, you align with a vegan and eco-conscious approach while still achieving a natural sweetness in your smoothie bowl. This choice supports sustainable agricultural practices and ensures that you're consuming a product that is both ethically sourced and beneficial to your health. Enjoy the blend of flavors and the peace of mind that comes with making mindful, health-conscious choices.

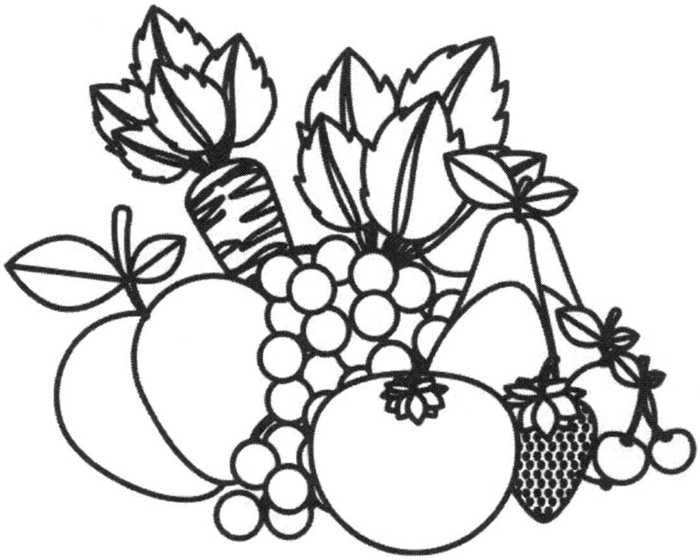

Avocado Toast to Boast: Elevate Your Breakfast Game

Bread has always held a special place in my heart—it's my first love. The comfort and warmth of freshly baked bread evoke memories of home and family. Yet, as much as I adore bread, not all varieties are created equal. It's crucial to choose the right kind to support both flavor and health.

Why White Bread Falls Short: White bread, often made from refined flour, is stripped of most of its natural nutrients and fiber during processing. This type of bread rapidly converts into sugar in the bloodstream, causing quick spikes in blood sugar levels. Over time, frequent consumption of white bread can contribute to insulin resistance, weight gain, and increased risk of chronic conditions such as type 2 diabetes and heart disease. Additionally, its high glycemic index can lead to energy crashes and cravings, creating a cycle of unhealthy eating.

The Superiority of Organic Sprouted Bread: For bread enthusiasts like me, organic sprouted bread is the gold standard. Unlike conventional white bread, sprouted bread is made from whole grains that have begun to sprout. This natural process enhances the bread's nutritional profile significantly. Sprouted grains contain higher levels of essential vitamins (such as B vitamins), minerals (like magnesium and zinc), and antioxidants. They also offer increased fiber content, which aids in digestion and helps maintain stable blood sugar levels. Additionally, sprouted bread is easier to digest and is less likely to cause bloating or discomfort compared to refined white bread. The complex flavors and textures of sprouted bread also make it a more satisfying choice.

The Magic of Organic Avocados: When it comes to avocado toast, the quality of the avocado matters just as much. Organic avocados are grown without synthetic pesticides and fertilizers, making them a cleaner, more eco-friendly choice. These avocados boast a creamy texture and rich, buttery flavor that perfectly complements the toast. Choosing organic ensures that you're avoiding harmful chemicals and supporting sustainable farming practices.

How to Ripen Avocados: Ripening avocados can be a bit of an art. To ripen an avocado, place it in a paper bag at room temperature. The bag traps ethylene gas, a natural ripening agent released by the avocado, which speeds up the ripening process. For a faster result, you can add an apple or banana to the bag, as they also release ethylene gas. Once the avocado is ripe, you can store it in the refrigerator to slow down further ripening. Check it daily to ensure it doesn't become overripe.

Understanding Black Avocados: An avocado that turns black or develops dark spots may be overripe or starting to spoil. If the avocado is mushy and has a strong odor, it's best to discard it. However, if it's just a bit darker than usual but still firm, it might still be usable. Look for any off-putting smells or mold to determine if it's safe to eat.

Creative Uses for Overripe Avocados:

- **Smoothies:** Blend overripe avocados into smoothies for a rich, creamy texture. They add healthy fats and nutrients while enhancing the smoothie's richness.
- **Face Mask:** Overripe avocados can be used as a hydrating face mask. Simply mash them and apply to your face for a moisturizing treatment that soothes and revitalizes your skin.
- **Guacamole:** Incorporate overripe avocados into guacamole or other dips. The creamy texture will blend seamlessly with other ingredients, making for a deliciously rich dip.
- **Baking:** Use mashed overripe avocados in baking recipes like brownies or muffins. They add moisture and healthy fats, contributing to a tender texture in baked goods.

With these tips and insights, you can fully enjoy the delicious simplicity of avocado toast while making informed choices about the bread and avocados you use. This recipe not only celebrates the love of good bread but also promotes a healthier, more mindful approach to enjoying one of my favorite breakfasts.

Avocado Toast

Ingredients

- 2 slices of whole-grain bread (or your preferred bread)
- 1 ripe avocado
- Salt and pepper to taste
- Red pepper flakes (optional, for some heat)
- Lemon juice (optional, to prevent avocado from browning)
- Sliced tomatoes (optional)
- Fresh cilantro or parsley leaves (optional, for garnish)

Instructions

1. Toast the slices of whole-grain bread until they reach your desired level of crispiness.
2. While the bread is toasting, cut the ripe avocado in half and remove the pit.
3. Scoop the avocado flesh into a bowl using a spoon.
4. Using a fork, mash the avocado in the bowl until it reaches your preferred level of creaminess. You can leave it slightly chunky or make it perfectly smooth.
5. Season the mashed avocado with a pinch of salt and pepper to taste. Add a dash of red pepper flakes if you like some heat.
6. Once the bread is toasted, spread the mashed avocado evenly on each slice.
7. If desired, squeeze a bit of fresh lemon juice over the avocado to enhance the flavor and prevent browning.
8. Top the avocado toast with slices of tomato for extra freshness and flavor.
9. If you like, garnish your avocado toast with fresh cilantro or parsley leaves for a burst of color and added freshness.

Whether you're enjoying it as a quick, energizing breakfast, a nourishing mid-morning snack, or a light yet flavorful lunch, this recipe provides a delightful burst of creamy avocado goodness. The creamy texture of the ripe avocado pairs perfectly with the crisp, toasted bread, creating a harmonious balance of flavors and textures.

This recipe also offers endless customization possibilities to suit your personal preferences. Add a sprinkle of sea salt and freshly ground black pepper for a classic touch, or experiment with a variety of toppings such as cherry tomatoes, radishes, or a sprinkle of red pepper flakes for an extra kick. Fresh herbs like cilantro or basil can add a burst of flavor, while a drizzle of balsamic glaze or a squeeze of lemon juice can enhance the taste profile.

Enjoy the satisfaction of a meal that is not only delicious but also packed with nutritious benefits. Avocados are a rich source of healthy fats, fiber, and essential vitamins, making this toast a wholesome choice for a balanced diet. As you indulge in the delightful combination of creamy avocado, crisp toast, and your favorite fresh toppings, you'll appreciate both the simplicity and the elegance of this timeless recipe.

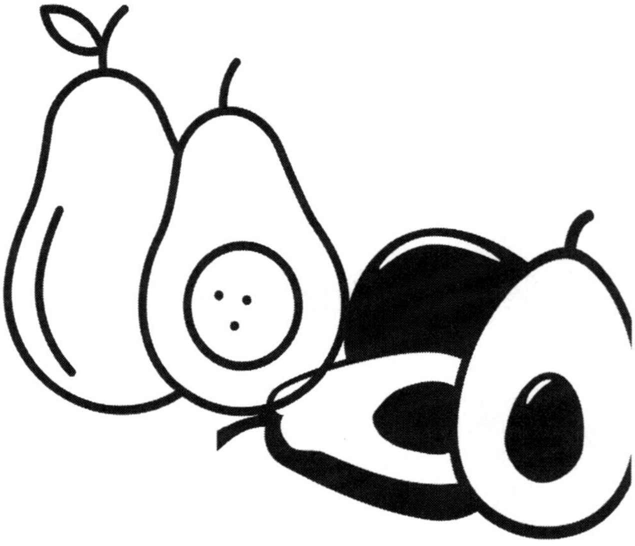

Pancake Paradise: Light and Fluffy Delights

Sunday mornings are a special time in our household, marked by the delightful aroma of fluffy pancakes sizzling on the griddle. My husband, a pancake enthusiast, eagerly anticipates this weekly tradition. It's a cherished ritual that brings comfort and joy to our weekends, and I've made it my mission to perfect the recipe to ensure every bite is as delightful as the last.

However, our journey to perfecting these pancakes has also led us to rethink some of our ingredients, particularly cane sugar. Cane sugar, a common sweetener, is linked to numerous health issues. When consumed in excess, it contributes to a range of illnesses including obesity, type 2 diabetes, heart disease, and dental problems. The rapid spike in blood sugar levels caused by cane sugar can lead to insulin resistance, which over time, increases the risk of developing chronic conditions.

Alternatives to Cane Sugar: To create a healthier pancake without compromising on taste, we've explored several alternatives to cane sugar:

- **Maple Syrup:** A natural sweetener with a rich flavor and lower glycemic index, making it a better option for maintaining stable blood sugar levels.
- **Honey:** Though not vegan, honey can be a natural alternative to cane sugar with its beneficial properties and lower glycemic impact. However, it should be used in moderation.
- **Stevia:** A plant-based sweetener with zero calories and no impact on blood sugar levels. It's a great option for those looking to reduce sugar intake without sacrificing sweetness.
- **Coconut Sugar:** Made from the sap of coconut trees, it contains some nutrients and has a lower glycemic index compared to cane sugar.

In our quest for healthier living, removing white bread, cane sugar, and other processed foods has had a profound impact. For instance, by eliminating cane sugar from our diet, my husband was able to manage and ultimately reverse his type 2 diabetes. This change, along with adopting a diet rich in whole foods and natural sweeteners, has significantly improved his health and well-being.

As you enjoy these fluffy pancakes, you'll appreciate how simple swaps can make a difference. We've incorporated healthier alternatives to ensure that every bite is not only delicious but also supportive of your overall health. Here's to savoring the perfect stack of pancakes, with the comfort of knowing they're made with thoughtful, health-conscious ingredients.

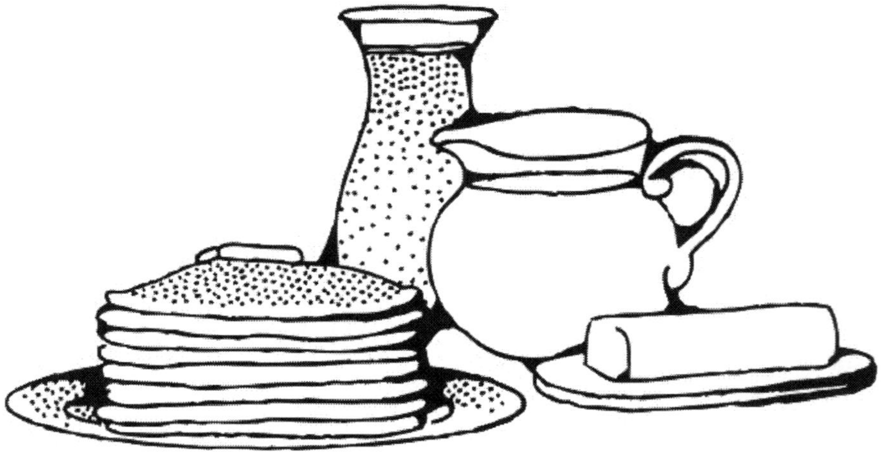

Fluffy Pancakes

Ingredients

- 2 cups unbleached organic all-purpose flour
- 2 tablespoons organic coconut sugar (or sweetener of your choice)
- 2 teaspoons aluminum free baking powder
- 1/2 teaspoon himalayan pink salt
- 1 cup plant-based milk (e.g., almond, coconut, or oat milk)
- 2 tablespoons melted coconut oil
- 1 teaspoon vanilla extract
- 2 tablespoons unsweetened applesauce
- 1 over ripe mashed banana

Instructions

1. In a mixing bowl, whisk together the flour, sugar, baking powder, and salt.
2. In another bowl, combine the plant-based milk, coconut oil, vanilla extract, and applesauce.
3. Pour the wet ingredients into the dry ingredients and stir until just combined. Be cautious not to overmix; a few lumps are okay.
4. Heat a non-stick skillet or griddle over medium heat. Lightly grease it with coconut oil or organic grass fed butter.
5. Pour a scoop of pancake batter onto the hot skillet, using about 1/4 cup of batter for each pancake.
6. Cook until bubbles form on the surface and the edges start to look set, typically 2-3 minutes.
7. Flip the pancakes and cook for an additional 1-2 minutes, or until golden brown and cooked through.
8. Transfer the cooked pancakes to a plate, and keep them warm while you cook the remaining batter.
9. Serve the vegan pancakes with your favorite toppings, such as maple syrup, fresh fruit, or dairy-free yogurt.
10. Enjoy your stack of fluffy vegan pancakes for a delicious and compassionate breakfast!

These fluffy pancakes are a delightful morning treat that will satisfy your cravings while aligning with your plant-based lifestyle. Whether enjoyed on weekends or as a quick weekday breakfast, they are sure to become a favorite in your kitchen.

When it comes to toppings, many people turn to butter for added richness. Organic grass-fed butter, which is made from the milk of cows exclusively fed grass, is valued for its rich flavor and enhanced nutrient profile, including higher levels of omega-3 fatty acids and vitamin K2. However, it's important to note that this butter is not considered vegan, as it is derived from animal milk. For those adhering to a plant-based diet, choosing plant-based butters or spreads made from oils and nuts is essential.

For those who enjoy experimenting with flavors, you can customize your pancake recipe by substituting bananas with sweet potatoes or even combining the two. Sweet potatoes can add a deliciously subtle sweetness and a creamy texture, while also providing additional nutrients such as vitamin A and fiber. To use sweet potatoes, simply cook and mash them until smooth, then blend them into your pancake batter. Combining sweet potatoes and bananas can create a unique flavor profile that enhances the pancakes' natural sweetness and adds depth to the texture.

By incorporating these healthy alternatives, you can enjoy pancakes that are both nourishing and delicious, all while staying true to your dietary preferences. Whether you choose to stick with bananas, opt for sweet potatoes, or combine them for a new twist, these pancakes are sure to delight and support your plant-based lifestyle.

Vegan Banana Nut Muffins: A Sweet and Nutritious Twist

Banana nut muffins are a beloved classic, celebrated for their sweet, moist crumb and the delightful crunch of toasted nuts. This vegan twist on the traditional recipe not only captures all the goodness of its non-vegan counterpart but also adds a compassionate touch by using plant-based ingredients. Whether you're a dedicated vegan or simply seeking a dairy and egg-free alternative, these Vegan Banana Nut Muffins are sure to satisfy your cravings for a comforting and flavorful treat.

One of the key ingredients in this recipe is nuts, which not only add a satisfying crunch but also pack a powerful nutritional punch. Nuts are rich in healthy fats, protein, and a variety of essential vitamins and minerals, including vitamin E, magnesium, and selenium. These nutrients support heart health, provide sustained energy, and contribute to overall well-being. By incorporating nuts into your diet, you're not only adding texture and flavor to your muffins but also boosting their nutritional value.

In my journey to create healthier recipes, I made a significant change by replacing cane sugar with coconut sugar in all my usual recipes. This decision was driven by the need to manage my husband's diabetes more effectively. Unlike cane sugar, which can cause spikes in blood sugar levels, coconut sugar has a much lower glycemic index, meaning it raises blood sugar more slowly and steadily. This makes it a better option for those looking to maintain stable blood sugar levels.

Coconut sugar is not only a healthier alternative to traditional sweeteners but also offers a natural, caramel-like sweetness that enhances the flavor of these muffins. It's far superior to artificial sweeteners, which often contain harmful ingredients. For instance, aspartame, a common artificial sweetener, has been linked to various health concerns, including headaches, dizziness, and even potential long-term neurological effects. By choosing coconut sugar, you're opting for a sweetener that's not only delicious but also better for your health.

These Vegan Banana Nut Muffins combine the wholesome goodness of ripe bananas, the nutritional benefits of nuts, and the natural sweetness of coconut sugar. The result is a muffin that's moist, flavorful, and guilt-free—a perfect start to your day or a satisfying snack anytime.

So whether you're making them for breakfast, a quick snack, or to share with loved ones, these muffins are sure to become a favorite in your home. Enjoy the taste of tradition with a modern, health-conscious twist.

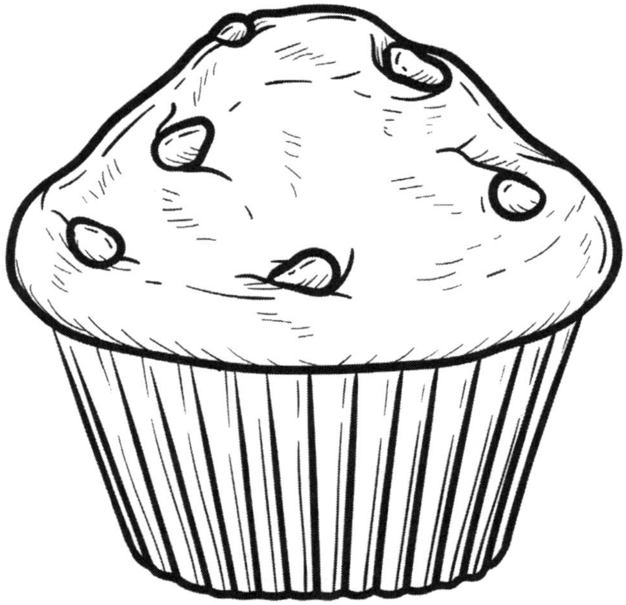

Banana Nut Muffins

Ingredients

- 2 ripe bananas, mashed
- 1/2 cup plant-based milk (e.g., almond, coconut, or oat milk)
- 1/4 cup melted organic coconut oil
- 1/2 cup organic coconut sugar
- 1 teaspoon vanilla extract
- 1 1/2 cups unbleached organic all-purpose flour
- 1 1/2 teaspoons aluminum free baking powder
- 1/2 teaspoon baking soda
- 1/2 teaspoon himalayan salt
- 1/2 cup chopped nuts (e.g., walnuts, pecans)

Instructions

1. Preheat your oven to 350°F (175°C). Line a muffin tin with paper liners or lightly grease the muffin cups.
2. In a mixing bowl, mash the ripe bananas until they're mostly smooth.
3. Add the plant-based milk, oil, coconut sugar, and vanilla extract to the mashed bananas. Mix until well combined.
4. In a separate bowl, whisk together the flour, baking powder, baking soda, and salt.
5. Pour the wet banana mixture into the bowl of dry ingredients. Stir gently until just combined. Be careful not to overmix; a few lumps are perfectly fine.
6. Fold in the chopped nuts and dairy-free chocolate chips (if using). This step adds delicious texture and flavor to the muffins.
7. Using a spoon or a scoop, divide the muffin batter evenly among the prepared muffin cups.
8. Bake in the preheated oven for approximately 20-25 minutes, or until a toothpick inserted into the center of a muffin comes out clean or with a few moist crumbs (but not wet batter).
9. Remove the muffins from the oven and let them cool in the muffin tin for a few minutes.
10. Transfer the muffins to a wire rack to cool completely. Once cooled, they are ready to enjoy!

Have you noticed that my recipes call for aluminum-free baking soda? This choice isn't just a matter of preference but a conscious decision to prioritize health. Aluminum, commonly found in conventional baking sodas and powders, can pose potential health risks. Studies suggest that excessive aluminum intake may be linked to neurological conditions such as Alzheimer's disease, as it can accumulate in the brain over time. By opting for aluminum-free baking soda, I aim to minimize these risks and ensure that the baked goods you enjoy are both healthier and safer.

Indulge in the deliciousness of these Vegan Banana Nut Muffins, a compassionate take on a classic favorite. With the irresistible combination of sweet, ripe bananas and the rich crunch of nuts, these muffins are perfect for breakfast, as a snack, or as a sweet treat any time of the day. Share them with friends and family, and celebrate the joy of cruelty-free baking!

For an extra burst of flavor and nutrition, consider adding fresh blueberries to your muffin batter. Blueberries are not only delicious but also packed with antioxidants, vitamins, and fiber. Their natural sweetness pairs beautifully with the bananas, and their juicy texture provides a delightful contrast to the nuts. Simply fold a handful of blueberries into the batter before baking to elevate your muffins and add a fruity twist that's both tasty and nutritious.

By making these thoughtful choices, you can enjoy your vegan muffins with enhanced health benefits and a burst of flavor. Each bite will offer a perfect blend of sweetness, crunch, and wholesome goodness, reflecting a commitment to both delicious and health-conscious baking.

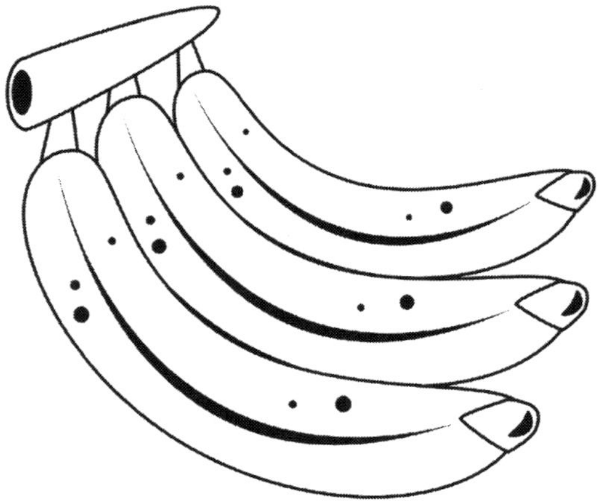

The Power of Seeds: A Nutritional Boost

The final breakfast recipe that I would like to share is Chia Pudding. This nutritious dish has become my workday go-to as it travels well and makes a convenient, healthy breakfast at the office. Its ease of preparation also makes it perfect for meal prep, allowing me to have a ready-to-eat, healthy option waiting for you in the fridge. Just grab and go!

Chia pudding is made with nutrient-packed chia seeds, known for their high fiber content, omega-3 fatty acids, and protein. By soaking the seeds in your choice of plant-based milk, you achieve a creamy texture that provides a satisfying and indulgent treat.

Chia seeds are a standout among seeds due to their impressive nutritional profile. These tiny powerhouses are packed with essential nutrients that can support overall health and well-being. Here are some of the notable benefits of chia seeds:

- **Omega-3 Fatty Acids:** Chia seeds are an excellent plant-based source of omega-3 fatty acids, which are crucial for heart health. Omega-3s help reduce inflammation, lower blood pressure, and improve overall cardiovascular health.
- **Fiber:** With a high fiber content, chia seeds support digestive health by promoting regular bowel movements and aiding in the prevention of constipation. Fiber also helps in maintaining healthy blood sugar levels and supporting weight management by providing a feeling of fullness.
- **Protein:** Chia seeds are a complete source of protein, containing all nine essential amino acids. This makes them an excellent option for those on a plant-based diet seeking to meet their protein needs.
- **Antioxidants:** Rich in antioxidants, chia seeds help combat oxidative stress and protect cells from damage. Antioxidants also play a role in reducing inflammation and supporting overall health.

What makes chia pudding truly special is its versatility. You can customize it with a variety of toppings, such as fresh fruits, nuts, seeds, and a drizzle of natural sweeteners like maple syrup or agave. This allows you to create endless flavor combinations and enjoy a new experience with each serving.

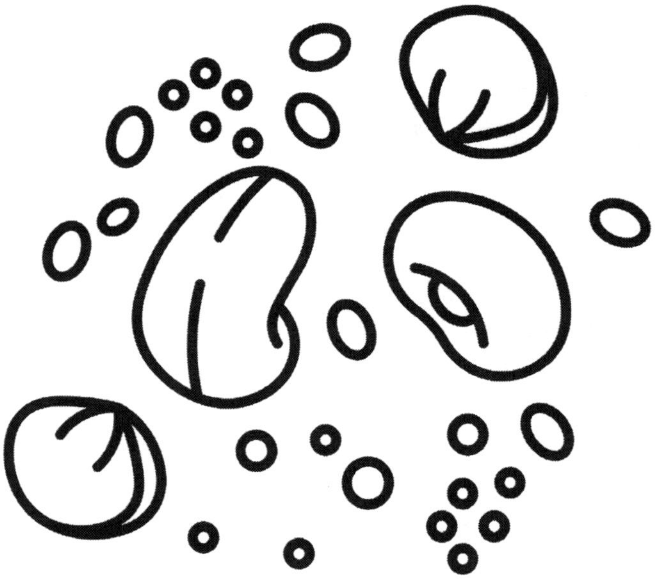

Chia Pudding

Ingredients

- 1/4 cup chia seeds
- 1 cup plant-based milk (e.g., almond, soy, or coconut milk)
- 1-2 tablespoons maple syrup or another sweetener of your choice (adjust to taste)
- 1/2 teaspoon vanilla extract (optional)
- Fresh berries, sliced fruits, or nuts for topping (optional)

Instructions

1. In a bowl, combine the chia seeds, plant-based milk, maple syrup (or other sweetener), and vanilla extract (if using). Mix well to ensure the chia seeds are evenly distributed.
2. Cover the bowl and refrigerate the mixture for at least 4 hours or overnight.
3. During this time, the chia seeds will absorb the liquid and create a pudding-like consistency. Stir the mixture a couple of times within the first hour to prevent clumping.
4. Once the chia pudding has thickened to your desired consistency, give it a final stir.
5. Serve the chia pudding in individual bowls or jars.
6. Top with fresh berries, sliced fruits, or nuts for added flavor and texture.
7. Enjoy your Vegan Chia Pudding as a wholesome breakfast, snack, or dessert.

As we reach the end of our chapter, it's essential to spotlight the incredible role seeds play in our daily diets. Seeds may be small, but they pack a nutritional punch that can significantly enhance your health. Adding seeds to your daily meals can provide a wealth of benefits, transforming ordinary dishes into nutrient-rich powerhouses.

Other Nutrient-Rich Seeds

In addition to chia seeds, several other seeds offer remarkable health benefits:

- **Flaxseeds:** Flaxseeds are another fantastic source of omega-3 fatty acids and fiber. They also contain lignans, which have antioxidant properties and may help reduce the risk of certain cancers. Flaxseeds can be added to smoothies, baked goods, or used as an egg substitute in vegan recipes.
- **Hemp Seeds:** Hemp seeds are rich in protein, containing all essential amino acids, making them a complete protein source. They also offer a balanced ratio of omega-3 and omega-6

fatty acids, which support heart health and reduce inflammation. Hemp seeds have a mild, nutty flavor that complement a variety of dishes.

- **Pumpkin Seeds:** Pumpkin seeds, also known as pepitas, are high in magnesium, zinc, and iron. These nutrients are essential for immune function, bone health, and energy production. Pumpkin seeds also contain antioxidants and healthy fats that support heart health and reduce inflammation.

- **Sunflower Seeds:** Sunflower seeds are a good source of vitamin E, an antioxidant that helps protect cells from damage. They also provide healthy fats, protein, and important minerals such as selenium and magnesium, which support overall health.

Incorporating these seeds into your diet can enhance the nutritional value of your meals and contribute to a balanced, healthful lifestyle. Whether you sprinkle them on salads, blend them into smoothies, or include them in baking, seeds offer a simple yet effective way to boost your intake of essential nutrients.

As we conclude this chapter with a focus on chia pudding, you can see how seeds like chia not only offer exceptional health benefits but also bring a delightful texture and flavor to your meals. Embrace the power of seeds and discover how these small additions can make a big difference in your health and wellness journey.

Mid-Day Delights

Here, in the heart of our culinary exploration, we arrive at a chapter that intimately understands the intricate dance of our busy lives. Midday, a time often overlooked in our relentless pursuit of daily goals, beckons us to pause, recharge, and indulge in a nourishing reprieve. This chapter is dedicated to those of us who navigate the tumultuous waters of packed schedules, demanding deadlines, and the ever-elusive lunch break.

As the sun climbs higher in the sky, we find ourselves caught in the ebb and flow of responsibilities, balancing the demands of our professional lives with our personal well-being. Lunch, once considered a fleeting interlude, becomes a precious moment—a chance to nourish not only our bodies but also our spirits.

Within these pages, we have carefully curated a selection of recipes that rise to the challenge of busy workdays. These dishes are a testament to the belief that even in the most hectic of schedules, one can find solace and delight in the midday meal.

Our culinary journey unfolds, inviting you to explore flavors, textures, and sensations that elevate the ordinary to the extraordinary. These recipes are tailored to seamlessly fit into your midday routine, promising not only sustenance but also a momentary escape from the demands of the outside world.

Join us as we embark on a voyage through the art of midday nourishment, discovering that even in the midst of chaos, there exists a sanctuary where flavors flourish and palates are pampered. Embrace this chapter as a testament to the idea that lunch, regardless of your bustling schedule, can be an oasis of culinary delight and rejuvenation.

Flavor Fusion: Chickpeas Meet Avocado

Introducing my first lunch recipe: Chickpea and Avocado Salad. This vibrant and nutritious dish showcases the incredible versatility and benefits of chickpeas, making it a perfect choice for a wholesome midday meal.

Chickpeas, also known as garbanzo beans, have a rich history dating back to ancient times. They originated in the Middle East and have been a staple in Mediterranean, Indian, and Middle Eastern cuisines for thousands of years. Today, chickpeas are enjoyed worldwide in a variety of dishes, from hummus and falafel to stews and curries.

Chickpeas offer numerous health benefits that make them a valuable addition to any diet. They are an excellent source of plant-based protein, fiber, vitamins, and minerals, including folate, iron, and phosphorus. Their high fiber content supports digestive health, while their protein helps build and repair tissues. Chickpeas also have a low glycemic index, which means they can help regulate blood sugar levels and promote satiety, making them an ideal ingredient for weight management and overall well-being.

In the realm of plant-based eating, chickpeas frequently serve as a replacement for meat, providing a hearty and satisfying texture to dishes. They are often used in veggie burgers, meatless meatballs, and as a protein-rich addition to salads and soups. Beyond meat substitutes, chickpeas have found their way into innovative culinary creations. Chickpea flour, for instance, is a popular gluten-free alternative used to make pizza crusts, pasta, pancakes, and even desserts like cookies and brownies.

This Chickpea and Avocado Salad combines the nutty flavor and firm texture of chickpeas with the creamy richness of avocados, creating a delightful and satisfying meal. Packed with nutrients and bursting with fresh flavors, this salad is not only delicious but also incredibly nourishing. Whether you're a dedicated vegan, exploring plant-based options, or simply looking for a nutritious and tasty lunch, this recipe is sure to become a favorite in your kitchen.

Chickpea and Avocado Salad

Ingredients

- 1 can (15 oz) organic chickpeas, drained and rinsed
- 1 ripe organic avocado, diced
- 1 cup organic cherry tomatoes, halved
- 1/2 organic cucumber, diced
- 1/4 organic red onion, finely chopped
- 2 tablespoons fresh organic cilantro, chopped
- Juice of 1 organic lemon
- 2 tablespoons organic expeller pressed olive oil
- Himalayan pink salt and pepper to taste

Instructions

1. In a large bowl, combine chickpeas, avocado, cherry tomatoes, cucumber, red onion, and cilantro.
2. In a separate small bowl, whisk together lemon juice, olive oil, salt, and pepper.
3. Pour the dressing over the salad and gently toss to coat all the ingredients.
4. Serve immediately, and enjoy your refreshing Chickpea and Avocado Salad!

In every forkful of this Chickpea and Avocado Salad, you'll discover a sensational blend of ingredients that transform a simple salad into a culinary masterpiece. Now, let's highlight one of the key ingredients: organic expeller-pressed olive oil. What is expeller pressed? Expeller pressing is a mechanical method of extracting oil from olives, which involves using a press to physically squeeze the oil out of the olives. This method is considered superior to traditional extraction methods because it doesn't involve the use of heat or chemicals, preserving the oil's natural flavor, aroma, and nutritional benefits.

Organic expeller-pressed olive oil is particularly prized for its purity and high quality. Unlike regular extra virgin olive oil, which can sometimes be extracted using heat or solvents, expeller-pressed oil ensures that the natural goodness of the olives is retained. This means more antioxidants, vitamins, and healthy fats in every drop, enhancing both the flavor and health benefits of your dishes.

Whether you're a dedicated vegan or simply exploring plant-based meals, this salad is a testament to the joy of wholesome eating. Prepare to savor the harmonious balance of flavors, textures, and colors in every bite, leaving you craving the experience long after your plate is empty.

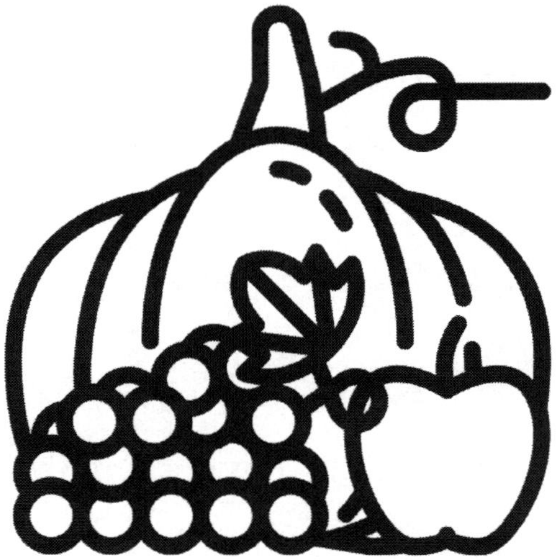

Caribbean Delight: Vegan Chickpea Curry

As someone of Caribbean descent who absolutely adores the rich flavors of curry, I want to share a delightful dish with you – Vegan Chickpea Curry. Curry isn't just a taste for me; it's a connection to my heritage, family gatherings, and the cultural celebrations that define who I am. In this recipe, I am honoring my Caribbean roots by infusing chickpeas with a medley of aromatic spices and creamy coconut milk, creating a curry that encapsulates the essence of the Caribbean.

Curry has a storied history, originating from the Indian subcontinent and spreading across the globe through trade, migration, and cultural exchange. In the Caribbean, curry has been embraced and transformed, becoming a staple in many households. The unique blend of spices used in curry powder often includes turmeric, coriander, cumin, fenugreek, and chili peppers, creating a symphony of flavors that tantalize the taste buds.

The Power of Turmeric

One of the key ingredients in our Vegan Chickpea Curry is turmeric. This vibrant yellow spice is not only essential for its earthy flavor and vivid color but also for its impressive health benefits. Turmeric contains curcumin, a powerful anti-inflammatory and antioxidant compound. Research has shown that curcumin can help reduce inflammation, improve brain function, and lower the risk of chronic diseases such as heart disease and cancer. It's also known for its ability to support joint health and promote a healthy digestive system.

The Caribbean Connection

In Caribbean cuisine, curry is often a cornerstone of many beloved dishes. The spices used in our Vegan Chickpea Curry are a nod to the traditional flavors that have been passed down through generations. The creamy coconut milk adds a luscious texture and a hint of sweetness that balances the spice, creating a harmonious blend that is both comforting and invigorating.

The preparation of our Vegan Chickpea Curry is straightforward, yet the result is a dish that feels complex and deeply satisfying. Start by sautéing onions, garlic, and ginger until they are soft and fragrant. Then, add the curry powder and turmeric, allowing the spices to bloom and release their flavors. Stir in the tomatoes and coconut milk, creating a rich and aromatic sauce. Finally, add the chickpeas and let the curry simmer until it thickens and the flavors meld together. For an added touch of nutrition, you can incorporate spinach or kale towards the end of the cooking process.

Enjoying the Dish

This Vegan Chickpea Curry is perfect for any occasion, whether it's a weeknight dinner, a family gathering, or a cultural celebration. Serve it over a bed of fluffy rice or with warm naan bread to soak up the delicious sauce. The combination of flavors and textures in this curry will transport you to the Caribbean, offering a taste of my heritage in every bite.

Embrace the rich traditions and health benefits of this Vegan Chickpea Curry, and let it become a cherished part of your culinary repertoire. Enjoy the vibrant flavors and the nourishing qualities of this delightful dish, knowing that you are honoring a time-honored tradition and promoting your well-being with every spoonful.

Vegan Chickpea Curry

Ingredients

- 1 can (15 oz) organic chickpeas, drained and rinsed
- 1 organic onion, chopped
- 2 cloves garlic, minced
- 1 can (14 oz) diced tomatoes
- 1 can (14 oz) organic coconut milk
- 2 tablespoons curry powder
- 1 teaspoon turmeric
- 1 teaspoon cumin
- Himalayan salt and pepper to taste
- Fresh cilantro for garnish (optional)
- Cooked wild rice or naan bread for serving

Instructions

1. In a large skillet, sauté the chopped onion and minced garlic over medium heat until the onion becomes translucent.
2. Stir in the curry powder, turmeric, and cumin, and cook for another minute until fragrant.
3. Add the diced tomatoes (with their juices) and coconut milk to the skillet, stirring to combine.
4. Bring the mixture to a simmer, then add the chickpeas. Let it simmer for about 10-15 minutes, or until the sauce thickens and the flavors meld.
5. Season with salt and pepper to taste.
6. Serve your Vegan Chickpea Curry over cooked rice or with naan bread, garnished with fresh cilantro if desired.
7. Enjoy a hearty and flavorful lunch with this delicious curry!

With each spoonful of our Vegan Chickpea Curry, you'll savor the vibrant flavors that speak to my Caribbean heritage and my profound love for curry. This dish is more than a meal; it's a journey that transports you to the heart of the Caribbean, creating memories and bringing joy to your table. Whether it's a regular weekday dinner or a special occasion, this curry is your chance to experience the richness of Caribbean cuisine and celebrate the shared love for flavors that transcend generations. Enjoy this culinary adventure!

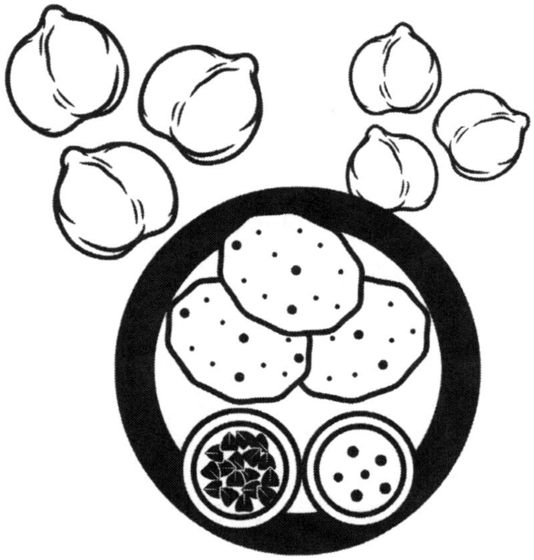

Stir-Fry Delight: Chickpeas, Garlic, Ginger, and More

When it comes to creating a nutritious and flavorful meal, our Chickpea Stir-Fry stands out as a delicious and healthful choice. This recipe not only showcases the versatility of chickpeas but also includes two powerful ingredients: garlic and ginger. Additionally, it features wild organic rice, or for a unique twist, it can be made with kelp noodles. Let's explore the health advantages of these components in detail.

The Healing Power of Garlic

Garlic, a staple in many cuisines worldwide, is renowned for its numerous health benefits. It has been used for centuries both as a food and as a medicine. Here are some key benefits of incorporating garlic into your diet:

- **Boosts Immune Function:** Garlic is rich in compounds like allicin, which has potent medicinal properties. It helps enhance the immune system, making it more effective at fighting off infections and illnesses.

- **Reduces Blood Pressure:** Studies have shown that garlic supplementation can significantly reduce blood pressure in individuals with hypertension. This makes it a natural remedy for maintaining cardiovascular health.

- **Lowers Cholesterol Levels:** Garlic has been found to reduce total and LDL cholesterol, which are risk factors for heart disease. Regular consumption can improve overall heart health.

- **Antioxidant Properties:** Garlic contains antioxidants that protect the body from oxidative damage. This can help prevent chronic diseases and support healthy aging.

- **Anti-inflammatory Effects:** The anti-inflammatory properties of garlic can help alleviate conditions like arthritis and promote overall joint health.

The Benefits of Ginger

Ginger is another potent ingredient with a long history of medicinal use. Its unique flavor and health benefits make it an essential addition to many dishes. Here are some of the benefits of ginger:

1. **Aids Digestion:** Ginger is known to promote healthy digestion by stimulating saliva and bile production. It helps alleviate gastrointestinal discomfort and is often used to treat nausea and indigestion.

2. **Reduces Inflammation:** Like garlic, ginger has powerful anti-inflammatory properties. It can help reduce pain and inflammation in conditions like osteoarthritis.

3. **Boosts Immune System:** Ginger's antioxidant and anti-inflammatory effects enhance the immune system, making it more effective at combating infections and diseases.

4. **Relieves Nausea:** Ginger is particularly effective at reducing nausea and vomiting. It's often used to alleviate morning sickness during pregnancy and motion sickness.

5. **Improves Circulation:** Ginger promotes healthy blood circulation, which can help prevent cardiovascular diseases and improve overall heart health.

The Superiority of Wild Organic Rice

Wild rice is a nutrient-dense grain that offers a range of health benefits. Unlike white rice, which is highly processed and stripped of many nutrients, wild rice retains its natural goodness. Here are some reasons to choose wild rice:

- **Rich in Nutrients:** Wild rice is an excellent source of protein, fiber, and essential vitamins and minerals, including magnesium, phosphorus, and B vitamins. These nutrients support overall health and well-being.

- **High in Antioxidants:** Wild rice contains more antioxidants than white rice, which can help protect the body from oxidative stress and reduce the risk of chronic diseases.

- **Low Glycemic Index:** Wild rice has a lower glycemic index compared to white rice, meaning it has a slower, more gradual impact on blood sugar levels. This makes it a better option for managing blood sugar and reducing the risk of type 2 diabetes.

- **Supports Heart Health:** The fiber content in wild rice helps reduce cholesterol levels and supports cardiovascular health. It also aids in digestion and promotes a healthy gut.

- **Naturally Gluten-Free:** Wild rice is naturally gluten-free, making it a suitable grain for those with gluten sensitivities or celiac disease.

The Benefits of Kelp Noodles

For a unique twist, you can substitute wild rice with kelp noodles in this recipe. Kelp noodles are made from kelp, a type of seaweed, and offer numerous health benefits:

1. **Low in Calories:** Kelp noodles are very low in calories, making them an excellent option for those looking to reduce calorie intake while still enjoying a satisfying meal.

2. **Rich in Nutrients:** Kelp is packed with essential nutrients, including iodine, which supports thyroid function, as well as vitamins A, C, and E, and minerals like calcium and iron.

3. **Gluten-Free:** Kelp noodles are naturally gluten-free, making them a great alternative for individuals with gluten sensitivities or those following a gluten-free diet.

4. **Supports Digestive Health:** The fiber in kelp noodles aids in digestion and helps maintain a healthy gut.

5. **Detoxifying Properties:** Kelp contains natural detoxifiers that can help cleanse the body of toxins.

Embracing a Wholesome Meal

In this Chickpea Stir-Fry, the combination of garlic and ginger not only enhances the flavor but also brings a wealth of health benefits to the dish. Paired with nutrient-rich wild organic rice or kelp noodles, this stir-fry is a powerhouse of nutrition and taste. Chickpeas provide a hearty source of plant-based protein and fiber, making this meal satisfying and nourishing.

Chickpea and Vegetable Stir-Fry

Ingredients

- 1 can (15 oz) organic chickpeas, drained and rinsed
- 2 cups mixed vegetables (bell peppers, broccoli, carrots, snap peas, etc.), chopped
- 1 tablespoon organic expeller pressed olive oil
- 2 cloves garlic, minced
- 1 tablespoon ginger, minced
- 3 tablespoons organic soy sauce (or tamari for a gluten-free option)
- 1 tablespoon organic maple syrup or agave nectar
- 1 teaspoon sesame oil (optional)
- Organic wild rice (cooked) or kelp noodles for serving

Instructions

1. In a small bowl, whisk together the soy sauce, maple syrup (or agave nectar), and sesame oil (if using). Set aside.
2. Heat oil in a large skillet or wok over medium-high heat. Add minced garlic and ginger, and sauté for about 30 seconds until fragrant.
3. Add the chopped vegetables to the skillet and stir-fry for 4-5 minutes, or until they start to become tender.
4. Stir in the drained chickpeas and the prepared sauce. Continue stir-frying for an additional 3-4 minutes until the sauce thickens and the chickpeas are heated through.
5. Serve your Vegan Chickpea and Vegetable Stir-Fry hot over cooked rice or noodles. Enjoy your flavorful and nutritious lunch!

In every forkful of this Vegan Chickpea and Vegetable Stir-Fry, you'll experience the harmony of textures and the explosion of flavors that make plant-based eating a true delight. This dish is a testament to the creativity of vegan cuisine, offering a nourishing and delicious lunch option. Whether it's a busy workday or a leisurely weekend, this stir-fry will leave you with a contented smile, knowing you've enjoyed a wholesome and satisfying meal.

Lentil Love: A Hearty Vegan Soup

Soup is the perfect meal for those with busy schedules, offering both convenience and nourishment. It's an ideal option for eating on the go, whether you're heading to work or packing lunch for your kids. One of the greatest benefits of soup is its ability to be prepared in large batches, making meal prep a breeze. Imagine spending a Sunday afternoon cooking a big pot of soup, then enjoying the fruits of your labor throughout the week. This approach saves time and ensures you have a healthy, homemade meal ready whenever you need it.

For those who work outside the home, soup can be a lifesaver. Simply store it in individual portions, and when it's time to head to the office, grab a container and heat it up for a delicious and satisfying lunch. Kids can also benefit from this easy meal solution. Pack their soup in a thermal container, ensuring it stays warm until lunchtime. It's a great way to provide them with a nutritious and comforting meal even when they're away from home.

Now, let's talk about the star ingredient of this recipe: lentils. Lentils are small, lens-shaped legumes that come in a variety of colors, including green, brown, red, and black. They have been a staple in many cultures for thousands of years, prized for their nutritional value and versatility in cooking. Lentils are incredibly nutritious, packed with protein, fiber, iron, and folate. They are also low in fat and calories, making them an excellent choice for those looking to maintain a healthy diet.

The health benefits of lentils are numerous. Their high fiber content supports digestive health and helps regulate blood sugar levels, making them beneficial for individuals with diabetes. Lentils are also a great source of plant-based protein, which is essential for muscle repair and growth. The iron in lentils helps combat fatigue and supports healthy blood cell production, while folate is crucial for brain function and prenatal health.

In addition to their nutritional benefits, lentils can be used in a variety of dishes. From soups and stews to salads and side dishes, lentils add a hearty and satisfying element to any meal. They absorb flavors well, making them perfect for incorporating into richly seasoned soups like our Vegan Lentil Soup.

This Vegan Lentil Soup is a delicious, warming, and nutritious option for anyone looking to enjoy a wholesome meal. Packed with vegetables, spices, and, of course, lentils, this soup is sure to become a favorite in your household. Whether you're meal prepping for the week or looking for a quick, healthy lunch, this soup has got you covered.

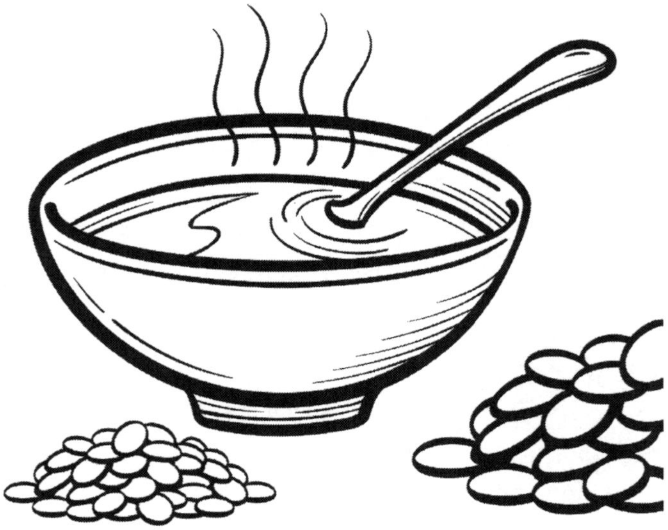

Vegan Lentil Soup

Ingredients

- 1 cup dried organic green or brown lentils, rinsed and drained
- 1 organic onion, chopped
- 2 organic carrots, diced
- 2 organic celery stalks, chopped
- 3 cloves garlic, minced
- 1 can (14 oz) diced tomatoes
- 6 cups organic vegetable broth
- 1 tablespoon of oregano
- 1 teaspoon cumin
- 1 teaspoon smoked paprika
- Himalayan pink salt and pepper to taste
- Fresh organic parsley for garnish (optional)

Instructions

1. In a large soup pot, sauté the chopped onion, carrots, and celery over medium heat until they begin to soften.
2. Add the minced garlic, oregano, cumin, and smoked paprika. Sauté for another minute until fragrant.
3. Stir in the lentils, diced tomatoes, and vegetable broth. Bring the mixture to a boil.
4. Reduce the heat to a simmer, cover the pot, and let it cook for about 25-30 minutes, or until the lentils are tender.
5. Season the soup with salt and pepper to taste.
6. Serve hot, garnished with fresh parsley if desired. Enjoy your hearty Vegan Lentil Soup!

As you savor each spoonful of this Vegan Lentil Soup, you'll experience the delightful marriage of earthy lentils, aromatic spices, and hearty vegetables. This nourishing soup is a testament to the comfort and satisfaction that plant-based eating can bring. Lentils provide a rich, protein-packed base, while the blend of spices adds depth and warmth to every bite. The fresh vegetables enhance the texture and flavor, creating a well-balanced and hearty meal.

This soup is perfect for anyone looking to enjoy a wholesome, delicious, and convenient meal. Whether you're a dedicated vegan or someone looking to embrace more meatless meals, this soup will leave you with a sense of warmth and contentment, making it a staple in your culinary repertoire.

Enjoy it fresh, or prepare a large batch to savor throughout the week. Its versatility and ease of preparation make it an excellent option for busy weekdays, and its comforting flavors make it a go-to choice for cold evenings. This Vegan Lentil Soup embodies the essence of nourishing, plant-based cooking and is sure to become a beloved recipe in your kitchen.

Harvest Delight: Quinoa & Roasted Veggie Bowl

If you are in the mood for something hearty and delicious, try this Quinoa and Roasted Vegetable Bowl. This dish celebrates the abundance and variety of vegetables, emphasizing the importance of incorporating a diverse range of produce into your diet. A colorful array of vegetables not only adds visual appeal but also ensures you receive a broad spectrum of nutrients essential for optimal health.

Vegetables are vital components of a healthy diet, offering numerous health benefits and helping to prevent various chronic diseases. The vegetables in this recipe, such as zucchini, spinach, and tomatoes, are nutritional powerhouses packed with vitamins, minerals, and antioxidants.

Spinach is one of the star ingredients in this bowl. This leafy green is incredibly nutrient-dense, providing a wealth of vitamins A, C, and K, as well as folate, iron, and calcium. Spinach is known for its high levels of antioxidants, which help combat oxidative stress and inflammation in the body. Consuming spinach regularly can contribute to improved eye health, thanks to its lutein and zeaxanthin content, which protect against age-related macular degeneration. Additionally, spinach supports bone health, boosts the immune system, and aids in maintaining healthy skin.

Tomatoes are another key component of this recipe. These vibrant red fruits are rich in vitamins C and K, potassium, and folate. One of the most significant compounds found in tomatoes is lycopene, a powerful antioxidant linked to numerous health benefits. Lycopene has been shown to reduce the risk of certain cancers, particularly prostate cancer, and to improve heart health by lowering LDL cholesterol levels and blood pressure. Tomatoes also have anti-inflammatory properties and support skin health, making them a valuable addition to any diet.

Zucchini is a versatile and low-calorie vegetable that adds a delightful texture to this bowl. It's an excellent source of vitamins A and C, manganese, and dietary fiber. Zucchini promotes healthy digestion, supports eye health, and helps maintain a healthy weight due to its high water content and low-calorie density.

The foundation of this bowl is quinoa, a nutrient-rich grain that has gained popularity as a healthier alternative to rice. Quinoa originated in the Andean region of South America, where it has been cultivated for thousands of years. It comes in various colors, including white, red, and black, each with a slightly different taste and texture.

Quinoa is a complete protein, meaning it contains all nine essential amino acids, making it an excellent protein source for vegans and vegetarians. It's also rich in fiber, magnesium, B vitamins, iron, potassium, calcium, phosphorus, and vitamin E. Compared to rice, quinoa has a lower glycemic index, which means it causes a slower, more gradual rise in blood sugar levels, making it a better option for blood sugar control. Its nutty flavor and fluffy texture make it a versatile ingredient in many dishes.

Incorporating a variety of vegetables and whole grains like quinoa into your diet can significantly improve your overall health and well-being. This Quinoa and Roasted Vegetable Bowl is not only delicious but also a nutritional powerhouse, providing a balanced meal packed with essential vitamins, minerals, and antioxidants. Enjoy the vibrant flavors and textures of this dish, knowing that each bite is contributing to your health and vitality.

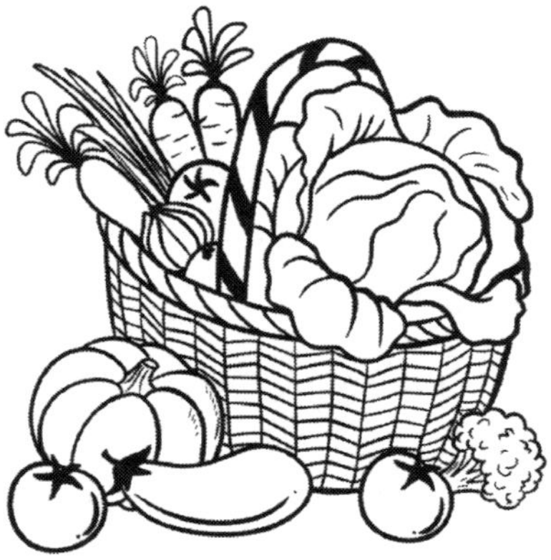

Quinoa and Roasted Vegetable Bowl

Ingredients

- 1 cup quinoa, rinsed and drained
- 2 cups mixed vegetables (spinach, zucchini, cherry tomatoes, etc.), chopped
- 2 tablespoons expeller pressed olive oil
- 1 teaspoon dried thyme
- 1/2 teaspoon garlic powder
- Salt and pepper to taste
- 1 diced organic avocado (diced)
- Fresh lemon juice for drizzling

Instructions

1. Preheat your oven to 400°F (200°C).
2. In a bowl, toss the mixed vegetables with olive oil, dried thyme, garlic powder, salt, and pepper.
3. Spread the seasoned vegetables on a baking sheet and roast in the oven for about 20-25 minutes, or until they are tender and slightly caramelized.
4. While the vegetables are roasting, cook the quinoa according to package instructions.
5. To assemble the bowl, divide the cooked quinoa among serving dishes, top with roasted vegetables, drizzle fresh lemon juice, and garnish with diced avocados.
6. Enjoy your Quinoa and Roasted Vegetable Bowl, a delightful and nutritious lunch!

In every spoonful of the Quinoa and Vegetable Bowl, you'll experience a fusion of tastes and textures that celebrate the essence of plant-based cuisine. This dish offers both nourishment and culinary satisfaction, making it a versatile addition to your menu. Whether you're a seasoned cook or new to meatless meals, this bowl exemplifies the joy of balanced, wholesome eating. Enjoy the flavors and embrace the health benefits of this delightful creation!

Mediterranean Manna Quinoa Salad

Since quinoa has so many health benefits, I wanted to share another household favorite quinoa recipe: Mediterranean Quinoa Salad. When I first introduced quinoa to my children, we often referred to it as "manna from heaven" due to its light, fluffy, and filling taste. The health benefits are an added bonus to its extraordinary flavor.

Quinoa, often dubbed a superfood, is rich in protein, fiber, and essential vitamins and minerals, making it a fantastic addition to any dish. It blends seamlessly into various dishes, enhancing their nutritional profile while delivering a delightful texture.

Our Mediterranean Quinoa Salad is a vibrant and refreshing dish that brings together the best of Mediterranean cuisine. The combination of quinoa, fresh vegetables, and flavorful herbs creates a salad that is both satisfying and nourishing.

Mediterranean Quinoa Salad

Ingredients

- 1 cup organic red quinoa, rinsed and drained
- 1 1/2 cups water or organic vegetable broth
- 1 cup organic cucumber, diced
- 1 cup organic cherry tomatoes, halved
- 1/2 cup organic Kalamata olives, pitted and sliced
- 1/4 cup organic red onion, finely chopped
- 1/4 cup fresh organic parsley, chopped
- 1/4 cup fresh organic mint leaves, chopped
- Juice of 1 organic lemon
- 3 tablespoons organic expeller pressed olive oil
- Himalayan pink salt and pepper to taste

Instructions

In a saucepan, combine quinoa and water or vegetable broth. Bring to a boil, then reduce the heat, cover, and simmer for about 15 minutes, or until the quinoa is cooked and the liquid is absorbed.Fluff the quinoa with a fork and let it cool to room temperature.

In a large bowl, combine the cooked quinoa, diced cucumber, halved cherry tomatoes, sliced Kalamata olives, finely chopped red onion, fresh parsley, and fresh mint leaves.

In a small bowl, whisk together the lemon juice, extra-virgin olive oil, salt, and pepper.

Drizzle the dressing over the quinoa salad and toss gently to combine, ensuring all the ingredients are well coated.

Taste and adjust the seasoning with additional salt and pepper if needed.

Serve your Mediterranean Quinoa Salad immediately, or refrigerate it for a refreshing and chilled dish. Enjoy the vibrant flavors of the Mediterranean!

As you savor each bite of this Mediterranean Quinoa Salad, you'll experience the magic of Mediterranean flavors, brought to life through a colorful and wholesome dish. This salad is a testament to the beauty of fresh ingredients and the delight of balanced, plant-based cuisine. Whether enjoyed as a standalone meal or as a complement to your dining experience, it's sure to leave you with a sense of vitality and satisfaction.

This Mediterranean Quinoa Salad is perfect for any occasion—whether it's a quick lunch, a side dish for dinner, or a potluck favorite. The combination of quinoa and fresh vegetables creates a balanced meal that is as nutritious as it is delicious. It's a testament to how wholesome ingredients can come together to create something truly special, providing both exceptional taste and numerous health benefits.

Bean There, Done That: A Corn and Black Bean Fiesta

When it comes to crafting a satisfying and nutritious salad, black beans and corn are a dynamic duo that truly shine. This Vegan Black Bean and Corn Salad highlights the incredible benefits of black beans, an ingredient that can effortlessly replace meat in many dishes traditionally made with ground beef. Here's an in-depth look at the origins, cultural significance, and health benefits of these fantastic components.

The Power of Black Beans

Origins and Cultural Significance Black beans, also known as turtle beans due to their hard, shell-like appearance, have been a staple in Latin American cuisine for centuries. They originated in the Americas and have been cultivated for thousands of years. Black beans are particularly prominent in Mexican, Cuban, Brazilian, and other Central and South American cuisines. They are celebrated for their rich, earthy flavor and their ability to absorb and complement a wide variety of spices and ingredients.

Nutritional Benefits

1. **High in Protein:** Black beans are an excellent plant-based protein source, making them an ideal meat substitute. They provide all essential amino acids, which are crucial for muscle repair and overall body function.

2. **Rich in Fiber:** The high fiber content in black beans aids in digestion, helps maintain healthy blood sugar levels, and keeps you feeling full longer, aiding in weight management.

3. **Packed with Vitamins and Minerals:** Black beans are a great source of vitamins and minerals, including iron, magnesium, folate, and B vitamins. These nutrients are essential for energy production, brain function, and overall health.

4. **Antioxidant Properties:** Black beans contain anthocyanins, powerful antioxidants that help protect the body from oxidative stress and reduce the risk of chronic diseases.

Soaking Fresh Beans for Enhanced Nutrition For those looking to maximize the health benefits, using fresh black beans and soaking them instead of opting for canned varieties is a fantastic option. Soaking beans overnight helps to reduce cooking time, improve digestibility, and enhance nutrient absorption. This process also helps in reducing the levels of certain antinutrients that can interfere with the absorption of minerals.

The Sweetness of Corn

Corn, another key ingredient in this salad, is not only delicious but also packed with nutritional benefits.

Nutritional Benefits

1. **Rich in Fiber:** Like black beans, corn is high in dietary fiber, which supports healthy digestion and helps regulate blood sugar levels.

2. **Vitamin and Mineral Boost:** Corn is a good source of essential vitamins and minerals, including vitamin C, thiamin (B1), folate, and magnesium. These nutrients contribute to immune function, energy production, and overall health.

3. **Antioxidants:** Corn contains antioxidants such as lutein and zeaxanthin, which are beneficial for eye health and may help prevent age-related macular degeneration.

Culinary Versatility Corn adds a natural sweetness and a pleasant crunch to the salad, enhancing the overall flavor profile. Its bright yellow kernels also add a vibrant color, making the dish visually appealing.

A Flavorful and Nutritious Combination

Combining black beans and corn in a salad creates a dish that is not only tasty but also incredibly nutritious. Black beans provide the protein and fiber necessary for a satisfying meal, while corn adds sweetness, crunch, and additional fiber. This salad can be a complete meal on its own or a hearty side dish.

Incorporating these ingredients into your diet can have a profound impact on your health. Whether you're a dedicated vegan or simply looking to include more plant-based meals in your diet, this Vegan Black Bean and Corn Salad is a testament to the delicious possibilities of wholesome eating. Enjoy the rich, earthy flavors of black beans combined with the sweet, crunchy texture of corn, and savor the health benefits with every bite.

Vegan Black Bean and Corn Salad

Ingredients

- 2 cans (15 oz each) black beans, drained and rinsed
- 2 cups sweet corn kernels (fresh or frozen, thawed)
- 1 cup bell peppers (red, yellow, or green), diced
- 1/2 cup red onion, finely chopped
- 1/4 cup fresh cilantro, chopped
- Juice of 2 limes
- 2 tablespoons olive oil
- 1 teaspoon cumin
- Salt and pepper to taste

Instructions

1. In a large bowl, combine the black beans, sweet corn, diced bell peppers, finely chopped red onion, and fresh cilantro.
2. In a separate small bowl, whisk together the lime juice, olive oil, cumin, salt, and pepper.
3. Pour the dressing over the salad and toss to combine, ensuring all the ingredients are well coated.
4. Let the salad marinate in the refrigerator for at least 30 minutes to allow the flavors to meld.
5. Serve your Vegan Black Bean and Corn Salad chilled as a hearty and refreshing lunch. Enjoy!

With each spoonful of our Vegan Black Bean and Corn Salad, you'll savor the Southwestern flair and the vibrant medley of ingredients that make this salad a true delight. This dish is a celebration of wholesome eating, offering both nourishment and culinary satisfaction. Whether enjoyed as a standalone lunch or as a side dish, this salad will leave you with a sense of vitality and a taste of Southwestern zest.

Savory Simplicity: Thai Peanut Noodle Bowl

Mid-day meals can often serve as the final meal of the day, especially if you're adhering to certain dietary practices or religious observances that involve skipping dinner. For those looking for a satisfying, nutrient-dense, and flavorful meal, this Thai Peanut Noodle Bowl is an excellent choice. The vibrant flavors of Thai cuisine are renowned for their complexity and balance, often featuring a harmonious blend of sweet, salty, sour, and spicy elements. Many Thai dishes naturally lend themselves to vegan adaptations, making them a favorite among plant-based eaters.

Some of the key ingredients in this Thai Peanut Noodle Bowl are bell peppers and cilantro, each bringing their unique benefits to the dish.

The Benefits of Cilantro

Cilantro, also known as coriander leaves, is a staple in many Thai dishes. It's not only loved for its fresh, citrusy flavor but also for its impressive health benefits:

Rich in Nutrients: Cilantro is a good source of vitamins A, C, and K, as well as folate, potassium, and manganese.

- **Antioxidant Properties:** The antioxidants in cilantro help protect cells from damage caused by free radicals.
- **Detoxifying Effects:** Cilantro is known to help the body eliminate heavy metals and toxins.
- **Digestive Health:** It aids in digestion and can help reduce bloating and gas.

Cilantro is also incredibly easy to grow at home. Whether in a garden or a small pot on your kitchen counter, cilantro can be grown in abundance, ensuring you always have fresh herbs on hand.

The Vibrancy of Bell Peppers

Bell peppers add a burst of color and a sweet, crisp texture to the dish. They come in various colors, including green, red, yellow, and orange, each offering unique nutritional benefits:

1. **High in Vitamins:** Bell peppers are packed with vitamins A, C, and B6. Red bell peppers, in particular, contain more than 200% of the daily recommended amount of vitamin C.
2. **Rich in Antioxidants:** They are a great source of antioxidants like carotenoids and flavonoids, which help reduce inflammation and protect against chronic diseases.
3. **Low in Calories:** Bell peppers are low in calories, making them an excellent addition to any weight management plan.

A Wholesome and Flavorful Meal

The Thai Peanut Noodle Bowl combines the benefits of cilantro and bell peppers into a delicious and satisfying dish. The noodles are tossed in a creamy peanut sauce, creating a flavorful base that is complemented by the fresh crunch of bell peppers and the bright notes of cilantro. This dish is perfect for lunch or an early dinner, offering a balance of flavors and nutrients that can sustain you through the day.

Thai Peanut Noodle Bowl

Ingredients

- 8 oz rice noodles (or any preferred noodles)
- 1 cup bell peppers (red, yellow, or green), thinly sliced
- 1 cup carrots, julienned
- 1 cup cucumber, thinly sliced
- 1/4 cup green onions, chopped
- 1/4 cup fresh cilantro, chopped
- 1/4 cup roasted peanuts, chopped (optional)
- Lime wedges for serving

For the Peanut Sauce

- 1/4 cup organic creamy peanut butter
- 3 tablespoons organic soy sauce (or tamari for a gluten-free option)
- 2 tablespoons organic maple syrup or agave nectar
- 1 tablespoon organic rice vinegar
- 1 clove garlic, minced
- 1 teaspoon ginger, minced
- 1/4 teaspoon red pepper flakes (adjust to taste)
- Water to thin the sauce (if needed)

Instructions

1. Cook the rice noodles according to package instructions, then rinse them under cold water and set aside.
2. In a small bowl, whisk together all the ingredients for the peanut sauce. If the sauce is too thick, add a bit of water to achieve your desired consistency.
3. In a large mixing bowl, combine the cooked rice noodles, thinly sliced bell peppers, julienned carrots, sliced cucumber, chopped green onions, and chopped cilantro.
4. Pour the peanut sauce over the noodle and vegetable mixture, tossing everything together to

ensure even coating.

5. Serve your Vegan Thai Peanut Noodle Bowl in individual bowls, garnishing with chopped roasted peanuts (if desired) and lime wedges. Enjoy your Thai-inspired noodle bowl!

As you indulge in each bite of our Vegan Thai Peanut Noodle Bowl, you'll be transported to the bustling streets of Thailand, where bold flavors and vibrant ingredients reign supreme. This dish exemplifies the global diversity of vegan cuisine, celebrating the unique and delicious plant-based options from cultures around the world—each bite of this noodle bowl brings the complex tastes of Thai cuisine, while nourishing your body with wholesome ingredients.

With the Thai Peanut Noodle Bowl, we bring our mid-day meals section to a flavorful close. Each recipe we've explored is a testament to the diverse and rich world of vegan cuisine, offering nourishing and satisfying options that celebrate the essence of plant-based eating. whether it's the aromatic spices of Thai food or the vibrant flavors of Caribbean dishes, or the rich tastes of Spanish cuisine. Enjoy the flavors, textures, and health benefits these dishes bring to your table, and continue to embrace the joy of global vegan cuisine.

The Significance of Dinner: A Time for Connection

Dinner, the heartwarming conclusion to the day's culinary journey, is a cherished ritual in cultures around the world. It's a time when we gather with loved ones, share stories, and replenish our bodies and souls with nourishment.

Dinner signifies more than just sustenance; it represents a culmination of the day's experiences, a chance to unwind, and an opportunity to choose foods that promote well-being. In this chapter, we delve into the significance of dinner and explore the delights of indulging in good, healthy vegan food as a central element of this evening tradition.

Dinner serves as a crucial pause button in our lives, offering a precious opportunity to reconnect with our families, friends, or even ourselves. It's a moment to set aside the hustle and bustle of the day, gather around a table, and engage in meaningful conversations. The act of sharing a meal promotes bonding, fosters communication, and strengthens relationships.

Beyond its social significance, dinner is a pivotal point in our daily nutritional intake. It's the last opportunity to fuel our bodies before a period of rest, making the choices we make during this meal particularly important. A well-balanced dinner can set the stage for a restful night's sleep, improved digestion, and overall health.

Eating Healthy Vegan Food: A Path to Vibrant Well-Being

Embracing veganism at dinner not only aligns with principles of compassion toward animals and environmental sustainability but also offers a multitude of health benefits. One key advantage is how our bodies process plant-based foods compared to meat.

Meat can take significantly longer to break down, which can negatively impact our health, especially when consumed late in the day. Eating meat late can disrupt our sleep patterns, cause digestive discomfort, and contribute to higher sodium intake, leading to elevated blood pressure. By eliminating meat from our diets, we can reduce blood pressure, improve digestion, and enhance overall sleep quality.

Furthermore, many prevalent illnesses are directly connected to our diets. Studies have shown that a diet high in processed meats and animal products is linked to an increased risk of chronic diseases such as heart disease, diabetes, and certain cancers. On the other hand, a vegan dinner plate brimming with colorful fruits, vegetables, legumes, and whole grains provides a rich array of essential nutrients, including vitamins, minerals, fiber, and antioxidants. These nutrients are vital for boosting our immune system, lowering the risk of chronic diseases, and promoting longevity.

The transition to a vegan dinner can also bring immediate and noticeable health benefits. Plant-based meals tend to be lower in calories and saturated fats, which can aid in weight management and reduce the risk of obesity-related conditions. Additionally, the high fiber content in plant-based foods promotes a healthy digestive system, preventing issues such as constipation and bloating.

In addition to the health benefits, vegan dinner options are incredibly versatile and flavorful. Contrary to misconceptions, vegan meals are far from bland or monotonous. They offer a world of culinary possibilities, with creative combinations of ingredients, spices, and cooking techniques that tantalize the taste buds and satisfy even the most discerning palate. Whether it's a hearty lentil stew, a colorful quinoa salad, or a spicy Thai curry, vegan dishes can be adapted to include the vibrant flavors of diverse cuisines from around the world.

Exploring vegan dinners allows us to experience the rich culinary traditions of various cultures while enjoying meals that are both delicious and nutritious. From the aromatic spices of Indian cuisine to the fresh, tangy flavors of Mediterranean dishes, vegan meals celebrate global diversity and the endless potential of plant-based cooking. Enjoy the journey of discovering diverse and delectable vegan dishes that nourish both the body and the soul.

In this chapter, we'll explore seven unique and delectable vegan dinner recipes that exemplify the joys of eating plant-based. Each recipe not only nourishes the body but also celebrates the diversity of flavors and textures that can be found in a vegan diet.

So, as we journey through the pages of this chapter, let's embrace the beauty of dinner—a time for connection, reflection, and the pleasure of savoring wholesome, vegan dishes that nourish both body and soul.

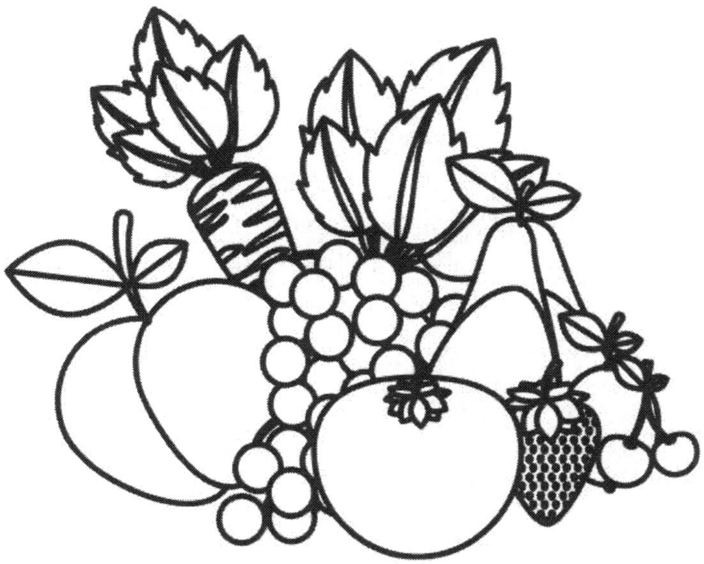

Healing Greens and Fruit Harmony

As we prepare to dive into our first dinner recipe, it's fitting to reflect on this scripture from Ezekiel. This verse beautifully captures the essence of nature's bounty, emphasizing the nourishing and healing power of fruits and leaves. It serves as a reminder of the incredible diversity and abundance of plant-based foods available to us.

When it comes to distinguishing between fruits and vegetables, it's common to encounter some confusion. Botanically speaking, fruits are the mature ovary of a flower and contain seeds, while vegetables encompass other plant parts, such as roots, stems, and leaves. Interestingly, many foods we commonly refer to as vegetables are actually fruits. For example, tomatoes, cucumbers, bell peppers, and zucchinis are all fruits because they develop from the flower of the plant and contain seeds.

In our upcoming recipe, we'll be using a delightful combination of leafy greens and fruits, celebrating the variety and versatility of these ingredients. Leafy greens, such as spinach and kale, provide essential vitamins, minerals, and fiber. These greens are also known for their healing properties: spinach is rich in iron and can help combat anemia, while kale is packed with antioxidants that support overall cellular health.

Furthermore, fruits like tomatoes and bell peppers add a burst of flavor and additional nutrients. Tomatoes, high in lycopene, are excellent for heart health, and bell peppers are loaded with vitamin C, boosting the immune system.

This dish not only aligns with the principles of plant-based eating but also honors the natural harmony between fruits and vegetables as highlighted in Ezekiel's vision. By incorporating these healing leaves and nourishing fruits into our diet, we embrace the full spectrum of nature's offerings, promoting both health and well-being. Prepare to experience the healing and nourishing power of nature's bounty in every bite.

Dinner is a crucial meal that should nourish and sustain us without weighing us down. Eating lighter meals in the evening allows our bodies to process and digest food more efficiently, preparing us for a restful night's sleep. Heavy meals, especially those rich in fats and proteins, can disrupt this process, leading to discomfort and impaired sleep quality. By choosing lighter, plant-based options, we promote better digestion and overall well-being.

This Spinach, Kale, and Fruit Salad with Bell Pepper and Cucumber is a perfect example of a light yet nutrient-dense dinner option. Packed with leafy greens like spinach and kale, this salad harnesses the healing power of greens. These leafy vegetables are rich in vitamins A, C, and K, as well as essential minerals like iron and calcium. They are known for their anti-inflammatory properties and ability to support heart health, improve digestion, and detoxify the body.

Fruits like apples, berries, and tomatoes add natural sweetness and a burst of antioxidants, which help protect our cells from damage and boost our immune system. The inclusion of fresh herbs and seeds further enhances the nutritional profile of this dish, offering a range of health benefits.

Leafy greens like spinach and kale are particularly beneficial due to their high chlorophyll content, which can help detoxify the liver and promote healthy skin. Additionally, these greens contain compounds that may reduce the risk of chronic diseases and support overall vitality.

Enjoy this Spinach, Kale, and Fruit Salad with Bell Pepper and Cucumber as a refreshing and nourishing evening meal that aligns with the principles of light, wholesome eating. Let the natural flavors and vibrant colors delight your senses while providing your body with the nutrients it needs to heal and thrive.

Spinach, Kale, and Fruit Salad with Bell Pepper and Cucumber

Ingredients:

- 2 cups fresh spinach leaves, washed and dried
- 2 cups fresh kale leaves, washed, dried, and chopped
- 1 cup cherry tomatoes, halved
- 1 bell pepper (any color), diced
- 1 cucumber, sliced
- 1 apple, cored and thinly sliced
- 1 avocado, diced (optional)
- 1/4 cup red onion, thinly sliced
- 1/4 cup fresh basil leaves, chopped
- 1/4 cup sunflower seeds or pumpkin seeds
- 1/2 cup blueberries or strawberries, sliced

Dressing:

1. 1/4 cup expeller pressed olive oil
2. 2 tablespoons balsamic vinegar
3. 1 tablespoon Dijon mustard
4. 1 garlic clove, minced
5. 1 tablespoon organic maple syrup
6. Pink himalayan salt and pepper to taste

Instructions:

1. Prepare the Ingredients:

- Wash and dry the spinach and kale leaves. Remove any tough stems from the kale and chop it into bite-sized pieces.
- Halve the cherry tomatoes, dice the bell pepper, slice the cucumber, and dice the avocado (if using).

- Thinly slice the apple, red onion, and strawberries (if using strawberries).
- Chop the fresh basil leaves.

2. Combine the Salad:

- In a large salad bowl, combine the spinach, kale, cherry tomatoes, bell pepper, cucumber, apple, avocado (if using), red onion, basil leaves, sunflower seeds, and blueberries or strawberries.

3. Make the Dressing:

- In a small bowl, whisk together the extra virgin olive oil, balsamic vinegar, Dijon mustard, minced garlic, maple syrup or honey (if using), salt, and pepper.

4. Dress the Salad:

- Pour the dressing over the salad and toss gently to combine, ensuring all the ingredients are evenly coated.

5. Serve:

- Serve immediately and enjoy the fresh, vibrant flavors of this nutritious salad!

This Spinach, Kale, and Fruit Salad combines the best of leafy greens and fruits, offering a perfect blend of flavors, textures, and health benefits. The addition of bell pepper and cucumber adds a delightful crunch, while the apple and berries bring a touch of natural sweetness.

As you may have noticed, all the recipes specifically call for pink Himalayan salt instead of iodized salt. This is due to the superior health benefits of pink salt.

Pink Himalayan salt is a pure, naturally occurring salt that contains over 80 trace minerals, including potassium, magnesium, and calcium. These minerals are essential for maintaining optimal health. Unlike iodized salt, which often contains additives and anti-caking agents, pink Himalayan salt is free from chemical processing and provides a cleaner, more natural taste.

Iodized salt, while fortified with iodine to prevent deficiencies, can be harmful when consumed in excess. It often contains synthetic additives that can disrupt the body's natural balance and contribute to health issues like hypertension and thyroid problems. Pink Himalayan salt helps regulate hydration, balance pH levels, and support healthy blood pressure without the unwanted additives.

Organic vs. Inorganic: Navigating Your Choices for Healthier Eating

When it comes to choosing between organic and inorganic foods, the decision can often come down to cost. Organic produce is typically more expensive due to the more labor-intensive farming practices and the lack of synthetic pesticides and fertilizers. However, it's important to remember that consuming healthy fruits and vegetables, even if they are not organic, is always a better option than eating meat, which can cause health issues and create toxins in the body over time.

Organic vs. Inorganic Produce: Understanding the Difference

Organic foods are grown without synthetic pesticides, fertilizers, and genetically modified organisms (GMOs). They are also free from artificial additives and preservatives. Studies have shown that organic produce can have higher levels of certain nutrients, such as antioxidants, compared to inorganic produce. For example, a study published in the British Journal of Nutrition found that organic crops contain up to 60% more key antioxidants than their non-organic counterparts.

In contrast, inorganic foods are grown using conventional farming methods that often involve synthetic chemicals and GMOs. While these practices can lead to higher yields and lower costs, they may also leave residues of pesticides and other harmful substances on the food.

Cost Considerations and Making Healthier Choices

While organic foods are often seen as the gold standard, their higher cost can be a barrier for many people. If price is an issue, it's still better to consume non-organic fruits and vegetables than to rely on meat, which can contribute to various health problems. Diets high in red and processed meats are linked to an increased risk of colorectal cancer. Additionally, meat can introduce toxins and unhealthy fats into the body, which can lead to heart disease, obesity, and other chronic conditions. It's crucial to emphasize that many of the diagnoses we face can be reversed by eliminating meat from our diets.

Homegrown Produce: An Affordable and Healthier Alternative

One of the best ways to ensure you are consuming healthy produce without breaking the bank is to grow your own fruits and vegetables. Home gardening allows you to control what goes into your food, ensuring it's free from harmful chemicals. It's also a cost-effective way to enjoy fresh, nutritious produce year-round.

Starting a home garden doesn't require a lot of space or resources. Many fruits and vegetables can be grown in small backyard plots or even in containers on a balcony or windowsill.

The Importance of a Lighter Dinner

Eating a lighter meal for dinner is crucial for several reasons. Our bodies' metabolic rate slows down in the evening, meaning heavy meals can be harder to digest and may lead to weight gain and discomfort. A study published in the journal *Appetite* found that consuming large meals late in the day can negatively affect blood sugar levels and insulin sensitivity, which can increase the risk of type 2 diabetes.

Instead, lunch can be the heaviest meal of the day, providing you with the energy you need to stay active throughout the afternoon. For dinner, lighter options such as salads, soups, or vegetable-based dishes are recommended. Skipping dinner altogether can also have its benefits. Intermittent fasting, which includes skipping meals like dinner, has been shown to improve metabolic health, reduce inflammation, and promote weight loss.

Pass the plate - Benefits of Skipping Dinner

Opting to skip dinner and replace it with a fruit or fruit and vegetable shake can significantly enhance your health. This practice is called intermittent fasting. Intermittent fasting is a dietary approach where you cycle between periods of eating and fasting. Intermittent fasting supports the body's natural repair processes and can lead to improved cardiovascular health, including reduced blood pressure and cholesterol levels.

Incorporating a nutrient-dense shake instead of a traditional meal helps improve digestion, increases energy, and can contribute to better sleep quality. This method not only aids in weight management but also supports overall metabolic health, making it a beneficial practice for enhancing well-being.

Regardless of whether you choose organic or conventional produce, focusing on incorporating more fruits and vegetables into your diet is crucial. Growing your own produce can be a fantastic, cost-effective alternative to store-bought options, offering both nutritional and financial benefits. By choosing lighter dinners or replacing them with nutrient-packed shakes, you support your body's health, promote efficient digestion, and improve overall vitality.

The Light Side of Dinner: Salads and Shakes for Better Well-being

Keeping in mind that dinner should ideally be light, opting for salads or shakes can be a game-changer for your health. My final dinner recipes focus on a combination of vibrant salads and nutrient-packed shakes designed to invigorate your evening meals without leaving you feeling overly full or sluggish.

These options not only provide a refreshing alternative to heavier fare but also support better digestion and overall well-being. By incorporating these lighter choices into your dinner routine, you'll enjoy a satisfying and health-conscious meal that won't weigh you down, ensuring a more restful night's sleep and promoting a balanced, vibrant lifestyle.

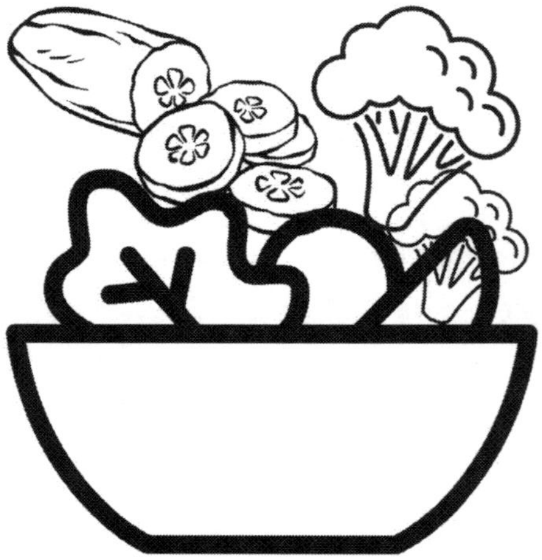

Citrus Avocado Salad - The benefit of Avocado

The Citrus Avocado Salad, is a delightful combination of fresh, vibrant ingredients that not only tantalize your taste buds but also provide numerous health benefits. This salad features the creamy richness of avocados and the zesty brightness of citrus fruits, creating a perfect harmony of flavors and nutrients.

Citrus Avocado Salad

- **Ingredients:**
  1. 2 ripe avocados, diced
  2. 2 cups mixed greens (arugula, spinach, and baby kale)
  3. 1 cup cherry tomatoes, halved
  4. 1/2 red onion, thinly sliced
  5. 1/4 cup toasted pumpkin seeds
  6. 1/4 cup crumbled feta cheese (optional)
  7. Dressing: Juice of 1 orange, 2 tbsp olive oil, 1 tbsp apple cider vinegar, salt, and pepper to taste
- **Instructions:**
  1. In a large bowl, combine the mixed greens, avocados, cherry tomatoes, and red onion.
  2. Sprinkle with toasted pumpkin seeds and crumbled feta cheese.
  3. In a small bowl, whisk together the orange juice, olive oil, apple cider vinegar, salt, and pepper.

4. Drizzle the dressing over the salad just before serving and toss gently.

The Benefits of Avocado

Avocados are often hailed as a superfood, and for good reason. They are incredibly nutrient-dense and offer a wide array of health benefits:

1. **Healthy Fats:** Avocados are rich in monounsaturated fats, particularly oleic acid, which is known to reduce inflammation and promote heart health.
2. **Fiber:** They are a great source of dietary fiber, aiding in digestion and helping to maintain healthy blood sugar levels.
3. **Vitamins and Minerals:** Avocados are packed with essential nutrients, including vitamins K, E, C, and B-6, as well as folate, magnesium, and potassium. These nutrients are vital for maintaining overall health, from supporting immune function to promoting healthy skin.
4. **Antioxidants:** They contain powerful antioxidants like lutein and zeaxanthin, which are beneficial for eye health.
5. **Satiety:** The combination of healthy fats and fiber in avocados helps keep you full longer, making them an excellent addition to any weight management plan.

The Power of Apple Cider Vinegar

This salad also incorporates apple cider vinegar (ACV) in the dressing, a time-honored ingredient celebrated for its medicinal properties. When choosing apple cider vinegar, it's crucial to opt for one that is organic and contains "the mother," a colony of beneficial bacteria that contributes to its health benefits.

1. **Anti-Inflammatory Properties:** ACV is known for its anti-inflammatory effects, which can help reduce symptoms of conditions like arthritis.
2. **Digestive Health:** The acetic acid in ACV can aid digestion by increasing the acidity of the stomach, which helps break down food more efficiently.
3. **Blood Sugar Control:** Studies have shown that ACV can improve insulin sensitivity and lower blood sugar levels after meals, which is particularly beneficial for those managing diabetes.
4. **Heart Health:** Regular consumption of ACV has been linked to reduced cholesterol levels and lower blood pressure, both of which are crucial for cardiovascular health.
5. **Weight Management:** ACV can promote a feeling of fullness, helping to reduce overall calorie intake.
6. **Menstrual Health:** Some women find that ACV helps alleviate menstrual problems, such as cramps and bloating, due to its potential ability to balance hormone levels.
7. **Detoxification:** ACV supports liver detoxification and overall body detox, which can enhance skin health and overall energy levels.

Incorporating just a tablespoon of apple cider vinegar from the mother into your daily diet, alongside a balanced vegan and organic diet, can yield significant health benefits. It can help reduce inflammation, manage menstrual issues, lower high blood pressure, and support overall well-being.

This Citrus Avocado Salad is not only a feast for the senses but also a powerhouse of health benefits. Enjoy this delightful dish knowing that you're nourishing your body with some of the best ingredients nature has to offer.

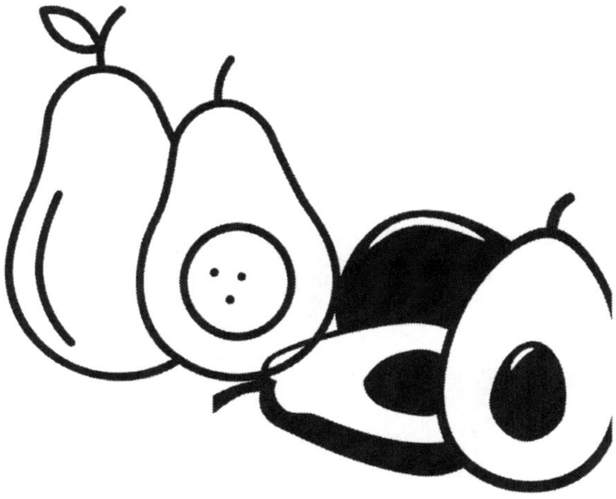

Popeye's Strength Salad: Spinach and Strawberry Fusion

Growing up, I vividly remember watching Popeye the Sailor, the cartoon character who would pop open a can of spinach whenever he needed an extra boost of strength to take on the bad guys. It was a fun and entertaining way to encourage kids to eat their greens—not to give away my age or anything! But the message stuck with me, and as it turns out, Popeye was onto something. Spinach really does make us stronger, and its benefits go far beyond what a cartoon could convey.

In this simple Spinach and Strawberry Salad, the sweet, juicy bursts of ripe strawberries perfectly complement the earthy, savory notes of fresh spinach, creating a harmonious blend of flavors that tantalize the taste buds with each bite.

Spinach & Strawberry Salad

1. Ingredients:

- 4 cups fresh spinach
- 1 cup sliced strawberries
- 1/4 cup sliced almonds
- 1/4 cup crumbled blue cheese (optional)
- 1/4 cup thinly sliced red onion
- Dressing: 2 tbsp balsamic vinegar, 1 tbsp honey, 2 tbsp olive oil, salt, and pepper to taste

2. Instructions:

- In a salad bowl, combine the spinach, strawberries, sliced almonds, crumbled blue cheese, and red onion.

- In a small bowl, whisk together the balsamic vinegar, honey, olive oil, salt, and pepper.
- Drizzle the dressing over the salad and toss gently to combine.

The Strengthening Power of Spinach

Spinach is a true nutritional powerhouse, and it's no wonder it was Popeye's secret weapon. Here's why spinach is so beneficial:

1. **Rich in Nutrients:** Spinach is loaded with essential vitamins and minerals, including vitamins A, C, and K, as well as folate, iron, and calcium. These nutrients are crucial for maintaining healthy skin, vision, and bones.
2. **Iron Content:** Spinach is an excellent source of iron, which is vital for producing red blood cells and transporting oxygen throughout the body. This helps improve energy levels and combat fatigue.
3. **Antioxidants:** Spinach contains powerful antioxidants like beta-carotene, lutein, and zeaxanthin. These antioxidants help protect the body against oxidative stress and reduce the risk of chronic diseases.
4. **Bone Health:** Vitamin K in spinach is essential for bone health, aiding in calcium absorption and bone mineralization.
5. **Anti-Inflammatory Properties:** The flavonoids and carotenoids in spinach have anti-inflammatory properties, which can help reduce inflammation in the body and lower the risk of inflammatory conditions.
6. **Heart Health:** Spinach supports heart health by helping to reduce blood pressure and improve arterial function due to its high levels of nitrates and potassium.

The Antioxidant Power of Strawberries

Strawberries are not only delicious but also packed with antioxidants that offer numerous health benefits:

1. **High in Vitamin C:** Strawberries are a fantastic source of vitamin C, an antioxidant that helps boost the immune system, promotes healthy skin, and aids in the absorption of iron from plant-based foods.
2. **Anthocyanins:** These are the compounds that give strawberries their vibrant red color and are known for their antioxidant and anti-inflammatory properties. Anthocyanins can help protect the body against oxidative stress and reduce the risk of heart disease.
3. **Fiber Content:** Strawberries are rich in dietary fiber, which supports digestive health, helps regulate blood sugar levels, and contributes to a feeling of fullness.
4. **Polyphenols:** These antioxidants help improve blood sugar control, reduce inflammation, and

lower the risk of developing certain chronic diseases.

5. **Anti-Aging Benefits:** The antioxidants in strawberries can help combat the signs of aging by neutralizing free radicals that cause cellular damage.

Combining these two superfoods in the Spinach and Strawberry Salad not only creates a delicious and refreshing dish but also provides a nutritional boost that can support overall health and well-being. The vibrant flavors and the incredible health benefits make this salad a perfect choice for a light and nutritious meal.

Enjoy this Spinach and Strawberry Salad, and let it remind you of the strength and vitality that Popeye celebrated, while also delighting in the sweet, antioxidant-rich strawberries that make this salad truly special.

Smoothie Essentials: Go-To Shakes for Every Day

Shakes can include a variety of ingredients like fruits, vegetables, protein powders, and non-dairy yogurts. Rather than detailing every shake recipe, I'll share some of my favorite go-to options.

It's important to highlight that using high-quality ingredients and investing in a high-quality blender are essential when incorporating shakes into your daily routine. A good blender ensures smooth, well-blended shakes, maximizing their health benefits and supporting your overall well-being.

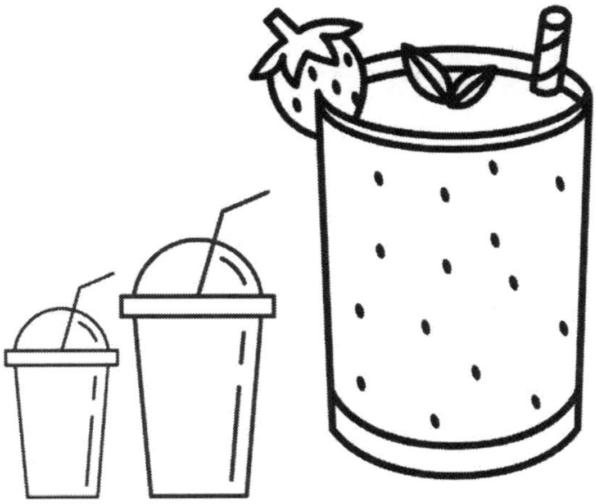

Green Detox Shake

- **Ingredients**
    1. 1 cup spinach
    2. 1/2 cucumber, peeled and chopped
    3. 1 green apple, cored and chopped
    4. 1/2 avocado
    5. 1 cup coconut water
    6. Juice of 1/2 lime
- **Instructions:**
    1. Combine all ingredients in a blender and blend until smooth.
    2. Pour into a glass and enjoy immediately.

Berry Beet Shake

- **Ingredients:**
    1. 1 cup mixed berries (strawberries, blueberries, raspberries)
    2. 1/2 cup cooked beetroot, peeled and chopped
    3. 1 banana
    4. 1 cup almond milk
    5. 1 tbsp chia seeds
- **Instructions:**
    1. Place all ingredients in a blender and blend until smooth.
    2. Serve chilled and enjoy the vibrant flavors.

Tropical Carrot Shake

- **Ingredients:**
    1. 1 cup pineapple chunks
    2. 1/2 cup carrot juice

3. 1/2 banana
4. 1/2 cup coconut milk
5. 1 tbsp flaxseeds

- **Instructions:**
  1. Blend all ingredients together until smooth.
  2. Pour into a glass and savor the tropical taste.

Creamy Kale and Pineapple Smoothie

- **Ingredients:**
  1. 1 cup kale, chopped (stems removed)
  2. 1/2 cup pineapple chunks (fresh or frozen)
  3. 1/2 avocado
  4. 1/2 cucumber, peeled and chopped
  5. 1 cup unsweetened almond milk (or any non-dairy milk)
  6. 1 tablespoon chia seeds
  7. 1 tablespoon flaxseeds
  8. 1 teaspoon spirulina powder (optional for extra nutrients)
  9. Ice cubes (optional, for a thicker texture)

- **Instructions:**
  1. Add the kale, pineapple, avocado, and cucumber to the blender.
  2. Pour in the almond milk and add the chia seeds, flaxseeds, and spirulina powder.
  3. Blend until smooth, adding ice cubes if desired for a thicker texture.
  4. Pour into a glass and enjoy immediately.

Benefits: *This smoothie combines the nutrient density of kale with the tropical sweetness of pineapple. Kale provides a rich source of vitamins A, C, and K, while pineapple adds digestive enzymes and a burst of flavor. The avocado contributes creaminess and healthy fats, while chia and flaxseeds boost omega-3s and fiber.*

Roasted Beet and Berry Smoothie

Ingredients:

1. 1 small roasted beet (peeled and chopped; can be roasted ahead of time and stored in the fridge)
2. 1/2 cup mixed berries (fresh or frozen; such as strawberries, blueberries, and raspberries)
3. 1 small banana
4. 1/2 cup unsweetened coconut yogurt
5. 1 cup unsweetened almond milk (or any non-dairy milk)
6. 1 tablespoon hemp seeds
7. 1 teaspoon honey or maple syrup (optional, for added sweetness)
8. Ice cubes (optional, for a thicker texture)

Instructions:

1. Place the roasted beet, mixed berries, banana, and coconut yogurt into the blender.
2. Add the almond milk, hemp seeds, and honey or maple syrup if using.
3. Blend until smooth, adding ice cubes if desired for a thicker texture.
4. Pour into a glass and enjoy immediately.

These dinner shakes are not only packed with nutrients but also offer a satisfying and flavorful way to end your day.

An Extra Dish to Complete Your Vegan Journey

Jamaican Jackfruit Oxtails: A Plant-Based Take on Tradition

When my oldest son was growing up, we often enjoyed what we affectionately called "linner"—a late lunch that seamlessly blended into an early dinner. One of his all-time favorite dishes was Jamaican style oxtails, and his excitement was always evident whenever I mentioned it. Since transitioning to a vegan lifestyle, I knew I couldn't write this cookbook without including his favorite recipe. So, I've recreated this cherished dish to ensure that when he visits for the holidays, I can still fill the house with the comforting aroma of his beloved meal. I saved the best for last, as a tribute to the wonderful memories we've shared around this comforting, hearty dish.

The History of Jamaican Oxtails

Jamaican oxtails are a beloved traditional dish with deep roots in the island's culinary history. Originally, oxtails were considered a less desirable cut of meat, often used by the lower classes. Over time, however, the resourcefulness of Jamaican cooks turned this tough cut into a tender, flavorful stew, rich in spices and slow-cooked to perfection. The dish became a staple of Jamaican cuisine, celebrated for its hearty and comforting qualities.

Transitioning to Vegan: From Oxtails to Jackfruit

After transitioning to a vegan diet, I sought to recreate the familiar and beloved flavors of Jamaican oxtails using plant-based ingredients. Jackfruit became the perfect substitute. Known for its fibrous, meaty texture, jackfruit mimics the mouthfeel of oxtails, making it an excellent alternative in vegan cooking.

Health Benefits of Jackfruit

Jackfruit is a powerhouse of nutrients and offers several health benefits that make it a superior choice to traditional oxtails:

1. **Rich in Nutrients:** Jackfruit is packed with vitamins A and C, potassium, magnesium, and antioxidants. These nutrients support immune function, skin health, and overall vitality.

2. **High in Fiber:** Unlike oxtails, which are high in saturated fat and cholesterol, jackfruit is low in fat and rich in dietary fiber. This helps with digestion, promotes heart health, and supports weight management.

3. **Low in Calories:** Jackfruit is naturally low in calories, making it a healthier option for those looking to maintain or lose weight without sacrificing flavor.

4. **Anti-Inflammatory Properties:** The antioxidants in jackfruit help reduce inflammation, which can lower the risk of chronic diseases.

Flavor and Texture

Jackfruit is not only nutritionally beneficial but also excels in mimicking the texture and flavor profile of oxtails. When cooked and seasoned properly, jackfruit absorbs the bold spices and seasonings used in traditional Jamaican oxtail recipes, offering a savory, slightly sweet, and tangy flavor. Its stringy, tender texture closely resembles the slow-cooked meatiness of oxtails, providing a satisfying and delicious alternative that honors the essence of the original dish.

By using jackfruit, I can enjoy the comforting flavors of Jamaican oxtails while embracing a healthier, plant-based lifestyle that aligns with my values and nutritional goals.

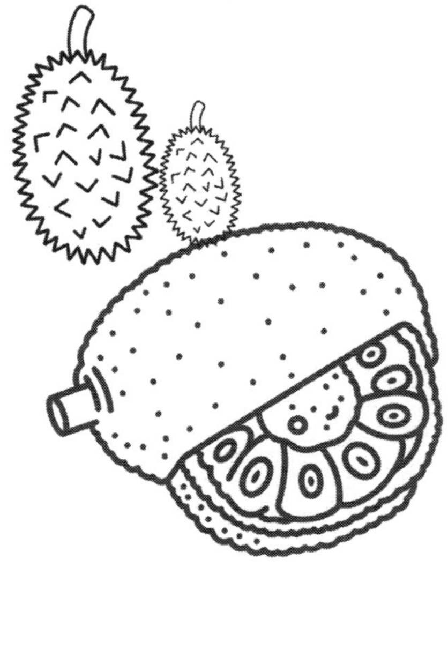

Vegan Jamaican Jackfruit "Oxtails"

Ingredients:

- 2 cans young green jackfruit in water or brine (organic, if possible), drained and rinsed
- 2 tablespoons organic coconut oil
- 1 large organic onion, chopped
- 3 organic garlic cloves, minced
- 2 organic scallions, chopped
- 1 organic Scotch bonnet pepper, chopped (remove seeds for less heat)
- 2 tablespoons organic soy sauce
- 1 tablespoon organic browning sauce (optional for deeper color)
- 1 tablespoon organic tomato paste
- 1 teaspoon organic dried thyme
- 1 teaspoon organic allspice (pimento)
- 2 cups organic vegetable broth
- 2 organic carrots, sliced
- 1 organic bell pepper, chopped
- 1 organic bay leaf
- 1 tablespoon organic coconut sugar
- 1/2 teaspoon himalayan pink salt (to taste)
- 1/2 teaspoon black pepper
- 1 can organic butter beans, drained and rinsed

Instructions:

1. Prepare the Jackfruit:

- Drain and rinse the jackfruit. Using your hands or a fork, pull the jackfruit pieces apart into shreds, leaving some chunks for texture.

2. Marinate the Jackfruit:

- In a large bowl, combine the jackfruit with soy sauce, browning sauce, dried thyme, allspice, and black pepper. Toss well to coat the jackfruit evenly. Let it marinate for at least 30 minutes (or overnight for deeper flavor).

3. Cook the Aromatics:

- In a large pot, heat the coconut oil over medium heat. Add the chopped onion, garlic, scallions, and Scotch bonnet pepper. Sauté until the onions are soft and translucent.

4. Add the Jackfruit:

- Add the marinated jackfruit to the pot, stirring to combine with the sautéed aromatics. Cook for about 5-7 minutes, allowing the jackfruit to absorb the flavors and slightly brown.

5. Add Tomato Paste and Vegetables:

- Stir in the tomato paste and cook for another 2 minutes. Add the carrots, bell pepper, and bay leaf, stirring to combine.

6. Simmer:

- Pour in the vegetable broth and add the coconut sugar and himalayan salt. Bring the mixture to a boil, then reduce the heat to low, cover, and let it simmer for 30-40 minutes, stirring occasionally.

7. Add Butter Beans:

- About 10 minutes before the dish is done, add the butter beans. Continue to simmer until the vegetables are tender and the flavors are well combined.

8. Serve:

- Remove the bay leaf and taste to adjust seasoning if needed. Serve the vegan jackfruit "oxtails" over a bed of steamed rice or with a side of your favorite Jamaican sides, like fried plantains or steamed cabbage.

This vegan version of Jamaican oxtails, made with jackfruit, offers all the savory, spiced goodness of the original dish while being a lighter and more health-conscious choice. The tender jackfruit soaks up the rich flavors of the spices and vegetables, making it a satisfying and comforting meal.

The End of the Journey: Savoring Every Moment

As we reach the end of this culinary journey together, we've explored a world of vegan delights that sustain and inspire us from dawn till dusk. From the wholesome breakfasts that start our days to the satisfying lunches, savory dinners, and what I lovingly call "linner," we've uncovered a wealth of plant-based treasures. These recipes are more than just dishes—they're cherished family traditions, adapted to embrace a vegan lifestyle.

Eating healthy and vegan is far from dull or monotonous. On the contrary, vegan cooking offers excitement and flavor as vibrant as any traditional meat-based meal. By choosing living, nourishing foods, we're energizing our bodies and supporting our well-being.

In these pages, I've shared my passion for plant-based eating and the beloved recipes of my family. Each dish reflects the flavors, traditions, and love that have graced our kitchen for generations.

As you bring these recipes into your own kitchen and onto your table, remember that vegan cuisine is a celebration of abundance and mindfulness. It's about appreciating the richness of plant-based ingredients, the joy of cooking, and the positive impact our choices can have on our health, the environment, and all living beings.

Beyond the delicious meals, consider the broader impact of your choices. Each plant-based dish you prepare is a step toward a more sustainable, compassionate, and healthful world. Your journey is helping to create a future where eating becomes an act of kindness, a celebration of flavor, and a testament to our shared responsibility.

Whether you're starting your day with a nourishing vegan breakfast, enjoying a fulfilling lunch, or relishing a delicious dinner, every meal is an opportunity to make a positive difference. Your choices and creativity are transforming your well-being and the world around you.

As you continue to explore vegan eating, may you find inspiration in the beauty of cruelty-free cuisine and the comfort of knowing you're part of a movement that embraces both the pleasure and responsibility of eating well. Savor these meals, and carry forward the traditions, flavors, and love passed down through the years.

With the knowledge and skills you've gained, you're ready to enjoy a week of vegan delights and beyond. This journey is just the beginning, filled with endless opportunities for discovery, compassion, and joy.

Bon appétit, and here's to a future where every meal celebrates health, harmony, and the vibrant flavors of the plant kingdom—recipes from my family's heart to yours.

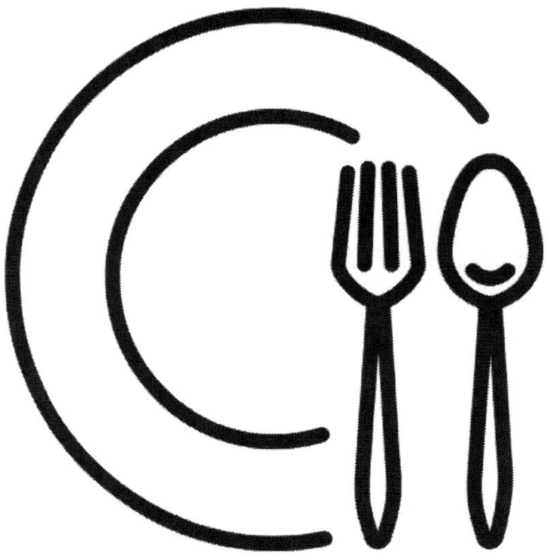

Jour Nique
Publishing Group

Made in United States
Orlando, FL
04 November 2026

90203419R00055